Sports Injuries of the Elbow and Hand

Guest Editor

WILLIAM B. GEISSLER, MD

HAND CLINICS

www.hand.theclinics.com

August 2009 • Volume 25 • Number 3

SAUNDERS an imprint of ELSEVIER, Inc.

W.B. SAUNDERS COMPANY
A Division of Elsevier Inc.

1600 John F. Kennedy Blvd. • Suite 1800 • Philadelphia, Pennsylvania 19103

http://www.theclinics.com

HAND CLINICS Volume 25, Number 3
August 2009 ISSN 0749-0712, ISBN-13: 978-1-4377-1223-0, ISBN-10: 1-4377-1223-1

Editor: Debora Dellapena

Hand Clinics (ISSN 0749-0712) is published quarterly by Elsevier Inc., 360 Park Avenue South, New York, NY 10010-1710. Months of publication are February, May, August, and November. Business and Editorial Offices: 1600 John F. Kennedy Blvd., Suite 1800, Philadelphia, PA 19103-2899. Customer Service Office: 11830 Westline Industrial Drive, St. Louis, MO 63146. Periodicals postage paid at New York, NY, and additional mailing offices. Subscription price is $282.00 per year (domestic individuals), $446.00 per year (domestic institutions), $144.00 per year (domestic students/residents), $321.00 per year (Canadian individuals), $510.00 per year (Canadian institutions), $383.00 per year (international individuals), $510.00 per year (international institutions), and $189.00 per year (international and Canadian students/residents). Foreign air speed delivery is included in all *Clinics* subscription prices. All prices are subject to change without notice. **POSTMASTER:** Send address changes to *Hand Clinics*, 11830 Westline Industrial Drive, St. Louis, MO 63146. Customer Service (orders, claims, online, change of address): Elsevier Periodicals Customer Service, 11830 Westline Industrial Drive, St. Louis, MO 63146. Tel: 1-800-654-2452 (U.S. and Canada). Fax: 314-523-5170. E-mail: journalscustomerservice-usa@elsevier.com (for print support); journalsonlinesupport-usa@elsevier.com (for online support).

Reprints. For copies of 100 or more of articles in this publication, please contact the Commercial Reprints Department, Elsevier Inc., 360 Park Avenue South, New York, New York 10010-1710. Tel.: 212-633-3812; Fax: 212-462-1935; E-mail: reprints@elsevier.com.

Hand Clinics is covered in *MEDLINE/PubMed (Index Medicus), Current Contents/Clinical Medicine, EMBASE/Excerpta Medica,* and *ISI/BIOMED.*

Printed and bound by CPI Group (UK) Ltd, Croydon, CR0 4YY

Transferred to Digital Print 2011

Contributors

GUEST EDITOR

WILLIAM B. GEISSLER, MD
Professor and Chief, Division of Hand and
Upper Extremity Surgery; and Chief, Section of
Arthroscopic Surgery and Sports Medicine,
Department of Orthopaedic Surgery and
Rehabilitation, University of Mississippi
Medical Center, Jackson, Mississippi

AUTHORS

MARK E. BARATZ, MD
Department of Orthopaedic Surgery, Allegheny
General Hospital, Pittsburgh,Pennsylvania

RANDY R. BINDRA, MD, FRCS
Professor, Department of Orthopaedic
Surgery, Loyola University, Medical Center,
Maywood, Illinois

MARK S. COHEN, MD
Professor and Director, Section of Hand
and Elbow Surgery; and Director, Orthopaedic
Education, Department of Orthopaedic
Surgery, Rush University Medical Center,
Chicago, Illinois

MATT CONTI, BS
Department of Orthopaedic Surgery, Allegheny
General Hospital, Pittsburgh, Pennsylvania

RANDALL W. CULP, MD, FACS
Professor, Department of Orthopaedic, Hand
and Microsurgery, Thomas Jefferson
University, Philadelphia; Philadelphia Hand
Center, King of Prussia, Pennsylvania

HOLGER C. ERNE, MD
Handchirurgie Rhoen-Klink, Handchirurgie
Rhoen-Klink, Saale, Germany

LARRY D. FIELD, MD
Director, Shoulder and Elbow Service,
Mississippi Sports Medicine and Orthopaedic
Center, Jackson, Mississippi

HABIMANA FONSECA-SABUNE, BS
Medical Student, Mount Sinai School
of Medicine, New York, New York

BRIAN J. FOSTER, MD
Resident, Department of Orthopaedic Surgery,
Loyola University Medical Center, Maywood,
Illinois

WILLIAM B. GEISSLER, MD
Professor and Chief, Division of Hand and
Upper Extremity Surgery; and Chief, Section
of Arthroscopic Surgery and Sports Medicine,
Department of Orthopaedic Surgery and
Rehabilitation, University of Mississippi
Medical Center, Jackson, Mississippi

JASON L. GOULD, MD
Resident, Department of Orthopaedic Surgery,
Mount Sinai School of Medicine, New York,
New York

DANIEL J. GURLEY, MD
College Park Family Care Center, Overland
Park, Kansas

MICHAEL H. HAUSMAN, MD
Lippman Professor; and Chief of Hand Service;
and Vice-Chair, Department of Orthopaedic
Surgery, Mount Sinai School of Medicine,
New York, New York

JENNIFER W. HSU, MD, MS
Resident, Department of Orthopaedic Surgery,
Mount Sinai School of Medicine, New York,
New York

JEFF W. JOHNSON, MD
Fellow, Philadelphia Hand Center, King
of Prussia, Pennsylvania; Adjunct Clinical
Assistant Professor, Department of
Orthopaedic Surgery, University of Arkansas
for Medical Sciences, Little Rock, Arkansas

ZINON T. KOKKALIS, MD
Orthopaedic Surgeon, Department of
Orthopaedic Surgery, Hand and Upper
Extremity Surgery, Allegheny General Hospital,
Pittsburgh, Pennsylvania

JEFFREY MARCHESSAULT, MD
Department of Orthopaedic Surgery, Allegheny
General Hospital, Pittsburgh, Pennsylvania

MATTHEW D. MILEWSKI, MD
Clinical Instructor of Orthopaedic Surgery,
Department of Orthopaedics and
Rehabilitation, Yale University School
of Medicine, New Haven, Connecticut

PERIKLIS A. PAPAPETROPOULOS, MD
Research Fellow, Hand, Upper Extremity and
Microvascular Surgery Training Program; and
Division of Orthopaedic Surgery, Department
of Surgery, Duke University Medical Center,
Hospital South, Durham, North Carolina

ANTHONY A. ROMEO, MD
Director and Associate Professor, Section of
Shoulder Surgery, Department of Orthopaedic
Surgery, Rush University Medical Center,
Chicago, Illinois

MELVIN P. ROSENWASSER, MD
Carroll Professor of Orthopedic Surgery and
Director of Hand and Orthopedic Trauma
Services, New York Presbyterian Hospital,
Columbia University Medical Center, New
York, New York

DAVID S. RUCH, MD
Director of Hand, Upper Extremity and
Microvascular Surgery Training Program; and
Professor of Orthopaedic Surgery, Division of
Orthopaedic Surgery, Department of Surgery,
Duke University Medical Center, Hospital
South, Durham, North Carolina

FELIX H. SAVOIE III, MD
Lee Schlesinger Professor of Orthopaedic
Surgery, Department of Orthopaedics, Tulane
University School of Medicine; Medical
Director, Tulane Institute of Sports Medicine,
New Orleans, Louisiana

SHANNON SINGLETARY, DPT, ATC, CSCS
Senior Associate Athletics Director; and
Certified Athletic Trainer; and Certified
Strength and Conditioning Specialist,
Department of Athletics, University of
Mississippi Medical Center, University of
Mississippi, Jackson, Mississippi

JOSEPH F. SLADE III, MD
Professor and Director, Hand and Upper
Extremity Service, Department of
Orthopaedics and Rehabilitation, Yale
University School of Medicine, New Haven,
Connecticut

DEAN G. SOTEREANOS, MD
Vice Chair, Department of Orthopaedic
Surgery, Hand and Upper Extremity Surgery,
Allegheny General Hospital, Pittsburgh,
Pennsylvania

IOANNIS C. ZOUZIAS, MD
Orthopedic Resident, Department of
Orthopedic Surgery, New York Presbyterian
Hospital, Columbia University Medical Center,
New York, New York

Contents

Preface   **xi**

William B. Geissler

The Emerging Role of Elbow Arthroscopy in Chronic Use Injuries and Fracture Care   **305**

Jennifer W. Hsu, Jason L. Gould, Habimana Fonseca-Sabune, and Michael H. Hausman

Arthroscopy is emerging as an invaluable tool for diagnosing and treating elbow pathology. In addition to the advantages of less scarring, decreased risk of infection, less postoperative pain, and a more thorough visualization of the elbow joint, arthroscopy is particularly well suited to the treatment of athletes trying to minimize rehabilitation and inactivity. Indications for elbow arthroscopy now extend well beyond diagnosis and loose body removal, and include the treatment of impingement, arthritis, contractures, fragment stabilization for osteochondritis dessicans, and treatment of certain fractures. This article reviews the basic principles and techniques of elbow arthroscopy and their application to common sports-related conditions, such as valgus overload syndrome, medial collateral ligament insufficiency, and the various causes of lateral elbow pain. Newer applications of elbow arthroscopy in fracture care are addressed as well.

Arthroscopic and Open Radial Ulnohumeral Ligament Reconstruction for Posterolateral Rotatory Instability of the Elbow   **323**

Felix H. Savoie III, Larry D. Field, and Daniel J. Gurley

Arthroscopic repair and/or plication of the radial ulnohumeral ligament (RUHL) complex can be as successful as open repair. The diagnosis of posterolateral rotatory instability (PLRI), made by a combination of positive clinical findings and radiologic evidence, can be confirmed by arthroscopic examination. The authors describe four clinical tests for PLRI. Magnetic resonance arthrography is recommended to assist in the preoperative evaluation. In surgical cases, the means to arthroscopically confirm instability are explained. Finally, the authors describe a repair and a ligament plication technique that can be performed by either arthroscopic or open technique with a high rate of success. Arthroscopic repair/plication of the RUHL is thought to effectively stabilize an elbow with PLRI, producing a high degree of patient satisfaction.

Open and Arthroscopic Management of Lateral Epicondylitis in the Athlete   **331**

Mark S. Cohen and Anthony A. Romeo

Lateral epicondylitis is the most common condition affecting the adult elbow. It occurs in middleaged individuals and is self-limiting in most cases. Based on clinical, histologic, and imaging data, the tendinous origin of the extensor carpi radialis brevis is the most likely site of pathology. When conservative measures fail, surgical management may be indicated. This can be accomplished by traditional open methods or by arthroscopic release. This article reviews the relevant anatomy of the common extensor tendon origin at the elbow and provides guidelines for surgical management of recalcitrant epicondylitis. Special emphasis is placed on arthroscopic techniques, which, when required, may allow for a more rapid return of the athlete to sport.

Medial Collateral Ligament Reconstruction in the Baseball Pitcher's Elbow   339

Holger C. Erne, Ioannis C. Zouzias, and Melvin P. Rosenwasser

Pitchers are prone to elbow injuries because of high and repetitive valgus stresses on the elbow. The anterior bundle of the medial ulnar collateral ligament (MCL) of the elbow is the primary restraint and is often attenuated with time, leading to functional incompetence and ultimate failure. Pitchers with a history of medial elbow pain, reduced velocity, and loss of command may have an MCL injury in evolution. Physical examination and imaging can confirm the diagnosis. Treatment begins with rest and activity modification. All medial elbow pain is not MCL injury. Surgery is considered only for talented athletes who wish to return to competitive play and may include elite scholastic and other collegiates and professionals. The technique for MCL reconstruction was first described in 1986. Many variations have been offered since then, which can result in predictable outcomes, allowing many to return to the same level of competitive play.

Biceps Tendon Injuries in Athletes   347

Zinon T. Kokkalis and Dean G. Sotereanos

Although rare, athletes involved in competitive strength training and contact sports may sustain distal tendon biceps injuries. Treatment of complete distal biceps tendon ruptures in athletes is primarily surgical. Early repair, through either one-incision or two-incision techniques with anatomic reinsertion of the ruptured tendon to the bicipital tuberosity, is highly recommended. In this article the etiology and pathophysiology of distal biceps tendon ruptures, current diagnostic modalities, and surgical indications are discussed. Also, treatment options, surgical techniques, outcomes, and potential complications are reviewed.

Arthroscopic Management of Scaphoid Fractures in Athletes   359

William B. Geissler

Fractures of the scaphoid are a common athletic injury. In this article the indications and treatment strategy for arthroscopic management of scaphoid fractures and non-unions in athletes are reviewed. Various arthroscopic assisted and percutaneous techniques for the fixation of fractures of the scaphoid are discussed, including the volar and dorsal percutaneous approaches, and arthroscopic reduction by the Geissler technique. In general, these techniques include a small amount of wrist arthroscopy and a significant amount of fluoroscopy.

Carpal Fractures in Athletes Excluding the Scaphoid   371

Jeffrey Marchessault, Matt Conti, and Mark E. Baratz

A wide range of hand and wrist injuries occur in today's recreational and elite athletes and account for 3% to 9% of all sports injuries. The onus is on the physician to discriminate between injuries that can be managed with an early return to sport, and those injuries that place the athlete at risk of further injury if they are not managed aggressively from the outset. The physician and the athlete must understand the balance between safe, early return to sport, and prompt surgical treatment that prevents late disability.

Repair of Arthroscopic Triangular Fibrocartilage Complex Tears in Athletes   389

Periklis A. Papapetropoulos and David S. Ruch

Triangular fibrocartilage complex (TFCC) injuries are a common source of wrist pain in athletes. These injuries constitute a unique orthopedic challenge because of the particular physical demands on these patients. A specialized management approach is often necessary, due to the short recovery time available and the need for high demand performances afterward. Arthroscopic repair of TFCC is becoming the treatment of choice in this group of patients.

Management of Carpal Instability in Athletes   395

Joseph F. Slade III and Matthew D. Milewski

Hand and wrist injuries are common in most athletic events and sports. Carpal fractures and ligamentous injuries are common in athletes and require physicians, trainers, and therapists who treat and diagnosis these injuries to have an understanding of the carpal bone anatomy and vascularity along with the potential for progression to instability. Research is still needed to further investigate the optimal treatments of all carpal injuries in athletes along with designing new means to prevent these injuries.

Operative Fixation of Metacarpal and Phalangeal Fractures in Athletes   409

William B. Geissler

Metacarpal and phalangeal fractures are common athletic injuries that can significantly affect the athlete's career when they occur during the season and affect the athlete's training when they occur in the off season. This situation is particularly relevant if there are complications or if fixation is not stable enough to permit early range of motion and rehabilitation. This article discusses percutaneous and open reduction techniques of hand fractures as these injuries pertain to athletes. The goal is stable fixation to allow early return to competition and rehabilitation.

Management of Proximal Interphalangeal Joint Dislocations in Athletes   423

Randy R. Bindra and Brian J. Foster

Proximal interphalangeal joint dislocations are common athletic injuries. In dislocations and fracture dislocations, the most important treatment principle is congruent joint reduction and maintenance of stability. This article reviews the relevant anatomy, injury characteristics, and treatment options for proximal interphalangeal joint dislocations and fracture dislocations. Treatment methods discussed include closed reduction, percutaneous fixation, and open reduction.

Acute Ulnar Collateral Ligament Injury in the Athlete   437

Jeff W. Johnson and Randall W. Culp

The functional thumb is a necessity for successful athletic participation. It not only allows the athlete to manipulate athletic equipment but also allows the precise manipulation of objects in the athlete's hand. Injury to the thumb often negates power grip and finesse of the athletic hand. Injuries can range from fractures, to dislocations, to ligamentous injuries. The relatively unconstrained thumb metacarpophalangeal joint is particularly vulnerable to injury from an abduction moment to its distal segment. Such injuries occur from direct contact and with falls on equipment such as racquet handles and ski poles. The stability of the athlete's metacarpophalangeal joint must be restored to allow for a productive return to sport.

Bracing and Rehabilitation for Wrist and Hand Injuries in Collegiate Athletes   443
Shannon Singletary and William B. Geissler

Athletic injuries of the hand and wrist are common. The key to management of these injuries is prevention. Certain sports require athletes to participate in positions that pose a higher risk of injury to the fingers and wrists. Once healing of the injured digit and wrist has occurred, rehabilitation of the injury is important. This requires close communication between the therapist and the strength and conditioning coach to allow strengthening exercises but limit traction to the involved injury in order to limit the risk of reinjury. Finally, once the injury has been rehabilitated, protective playing casts and splints are useful to allow the athlete to return early to competition and to decrease the risk of reinjury.

Index   449

Hand Clinics

FORTHCOMING ISSUES

November 2009

Hand Burns
Matthew B. Klein, MD, FACS,
Guest Editor

February 2010

Wrist Trauma
Steven Papp, MD, MSc, FRCS(C),
Guest Editor

May 2010

Complications in Hand Surgery
Jeff Greenberg, MD, *Guest Editor*

RECENT ISSUES

May 2009

Congenital Hand Differences
Kevin C. Chung, MD, *Guest Editor*

February 2009

Evidence-Based Practice
Robert M. Szabo, MD, MPH, and
Joy C. MacDermid, BScPT, PhD,
Guest Editors

November 2008

Nerve Transfers
Susan E. Mackinnon, MD, and
Christine B. Novak, PT, MS, PhD(c),
Guest Editors

THE CLINICS ARE NOW AVAILABLE ONLINE!

Access your subscription at:
www.theclinics.com

Preface

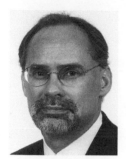

William B. Geissler, MD
Guest Editor

The incidence of athletic injuries continues to increase for a number of reasons. First, high school and collegiate athletes continue to grow in size, power, and speed as compared with the past. This results in higher velocity and energy injuries. In addition, "weekend warrior" athletic injuries continue to increase as our population continues to participate in athletic activities throughout the life span.

This issue of *Hand Clinics* concentrates on athletic injuries of the elbow, wrist, and hand. Previously, when one thought of athletic pathology, injuries to the knee and shoulder were usually first to come to mind. However, athletic injuries to the elbow, wrist, and hand are quite common, both in younger and older athletes. In the past mind set, these types of injuries to the upper extremity were trivial. Yet, if they are not ideally managed, complications can occur, which can keep the skilled athlete or weekend warrior out for a prolonged period of time.

Upper extremity experts from around the country offer their insight, tips, tricks, and pearls for management of upper extremity athletic injuries. The latest open and arthroscopic techniques involving injuries of the elbow, wrist, and hand are discussed in detail. In addition, the importance of rehabilitation and the early safe return of the athlete with protective bracing to competition are reviewed.

I would like to thank the internationally well-known authors for their contributions in the management of upper extremity athletic injuries in the hope of early safe return to athletic competition.

William B. Geissler, MD
Section of Arthroscopic Surgery
and Sports Medicine
Department of Orthopaedic Surgery and
Rehabilitation
University of Mississippi Medical Center
2500 North State Street
Jackson, MS 39216, USA

E-mail address:
3doghill@msn.com (W.B. Geissler)

Hand Clin 25 (2009) xi
doi:10.1016/j.hcl.2009.06.008
0749-0712/09/$ – see front matter

The Emerging Role of Elbow Arthroscopy in Chronic Use Injuries and Fracture Care

Jennifer W. Hsu, MD, MS[a],*, Jason L. Gould, MD[a],
Habimana Fonseca-Sabune, BS[b], Michael H. Hausman, MD[a]

KEYWORDS

- Elbow arthroscopy • Fracture • Tennis elbow
- Medial collateral ligament • Thrower's elbow
- Lateral epicondylitis

Arthroscopy is emerging as an invaluable tool for diagnosing and treating elbow pathology. In addition to the advantages of less scarring, decreased risk of infection, less postoperative pain, and a more thorough visualization of the elbow joint, arthroscopy is particularly well suited to the treatment of athletes trying to minimize rehabilitation and inactivity.[1] Indications for elbow arthroscopy now extend well beyond diagnosis and loose body removal, and include the treatment of impingement, arthritis, contractures, fragment stabilization for osteochondritis dessicans (OCD), and treatment of certain fractures.

This article reviews the basic principles and techniques of elbow arthroscopy and their application to common sports-related conditions, such as valgus overload syndrome, medial collateral ligament (MCL) insufficiency, and the various causes of lateral elbow pain.

ANATOMY AND PORTAL PLACEMENT

Before surgery, a thorough examination under anesthesia is performed using the mini-fluoroscope to check for congruous joint motion and valgus, posterolateral, or anterior instability.[2] Elbow arthroscopy can be performed in the prone, lateral decubitus, or supine positions. The lateral decubitus position is popular, although the senior author prefers the supine positioning using an arm holder (such as the McConnell arm holder; McConnell Orthopaedic Manufacturing Co., Greenville, Texas) to place the arm across the patient's chest for access to the posterior compartment or at the side for work in the anterior aspect of the elbow. This procedure allows the arm to be moved about and simplifies conversion to an open procedure, such as MCL reconstruction, if necessary (**Fig. 1**).

The major topographic landmarks, including the medial and lateral epicondyles, the radial head, the radiocapitellar joint, and the ulnar nerve are palpated and marked. The elbow is flexed and extended to confirm that the ulnar nerve avoids subluxation with flexion. Previous submuscular transposition of the ulnar nerve is an absolute contraindication to making a medial portal.[3] Placement of a medial portal after the anterior subcutaneous transposition is permissible only if the nerve can be clearly palpated and the portal can be placed, using blunt dissection techniques, at a distance from the nerve. Care should be taken throughout the procedure to avoid levering instruments and potentially crushing the nerve.[4]

A tourniquet is routinely used. Injection of the joint with saline distends the capsule, which displaces the neurovascular structures and increases the ease and safety of portal placement.

[a] Department of Orthopaedic Surgery, Mount Sinai School of Medicine, 5 East 98th Street, Box 1188, New York, NY 10029, USA
[b] Mount Sinai School of Medicine, 5 East 98th Street, Box 1188, New York, NY 10029, USA
* Corresponding author.
E-mail address: jennifer.hsu@mssm.edu (J.W. Hsu).

Hand Clin 25 (2009) 305–321
doi:10.1016/j.hcl.2009.05.009

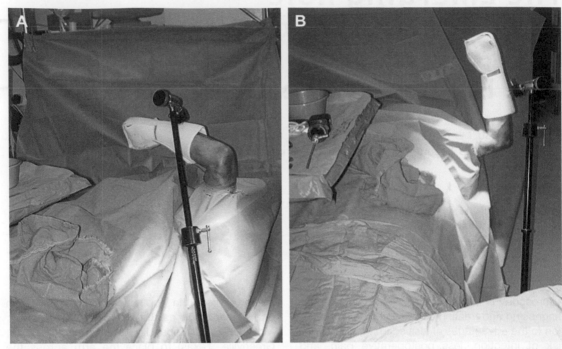

Fig. 1. The preferred patient positioning for elbow arthroscopy: supine with a McConnell arm positioner. (*A*) Position for access to the posterior compartment. (*B*) Position for anterior elbow access.

Low inflow pressure (25–30 mm Hg) is used to prevent fluid extravasation and soft tissue swelling. Retractors, rather than hydrostatic pressure, are used to increase exposure within the joint.[3]

The most commonly used portals include two medial portals, four lateral portals, and three posterior portals. Most of these portals are made by incising the skin with a #15 scalpel blade and bluntly spreading the subcutaneous tissues to protect the terminal branches of cutaneous nerves. Two exceptions to this are the transtriceps and posterolateral portals, which can be established with a #11 blade.

The two medial portals most commonly used are the proximal anteromedial and the anteromedial portals. The proximal anteromedial (or superomedial) portal is located just anterior to the intermuscular septum and 2 cm proximal to the medial epicondyle. The ulnar nerve, which lies 3 to 4 mm behind the septum, is at risk with this portal placement if it is placed too posteriorly[1,2] The anteromedial portal is established under direct visualization 2 cm anterior and 2 cm distal to the medial epicondyle, and is commonly placed to augment the proximal anteromedial portal when access to the medial recess is needed. The medial antebrachial cutaneous nerve lies 1 to 2 cm anterior and lateral to this portal, and is at risk for iatrogenic injury during placement. Portals should be made close to the capsular insertion on the supracondylar ridges, as capsular tissue trapped between the portal and humerus is not only difficult to access but also decreases the joint volume, thus compromising exposure (**Fig. 2**).[1]

There are four lateral portals used. The proximal anterolateral portal, located 1 to 2 cm proximal to the lateral epicondyle, provides accessory access to the medial recess of the elbow when instrumentation is required. The medial antebrachial cutaneous nerve is at greatest risk when establishing this route. The anterolateral portal is traditionally described as 3 cm distal and 2 cm anterior to the lateral epicondyle. The radial nerve is at risk of iatrogenic injury here. Moving the portal proximally into the sulcus of the radiocapitellar joint decreases this likelihood. The anterior radiocapitellar portal is slightly anterior and proximal to the radiocapitellar joint. As it lies closest to the radial nerve, direct placement should be made under direct visualization from a medial portal, and care should be taken to ensure that the trocar and cannula are not deflected anteriorly along the capsule toward the nerve. The direct lateral portal, or soft spot portal, is in the center of the triangle formed by the lateral epicondyle, olecranon process, and radial head. This portal allows visualization of the inferior capitellum and radioulnar articulation. During debridement of the posterior radiocapitellar joint through this portal, care

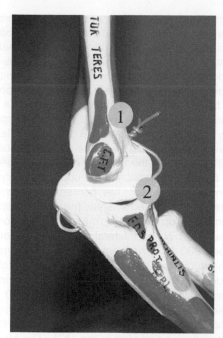

Fig. 2. A sawbones model of the medial elbow, relevant muscular origins/insertions, and the medial portals. (1) Proximal anteromedial/superomedial; (2) anteromedial portal.

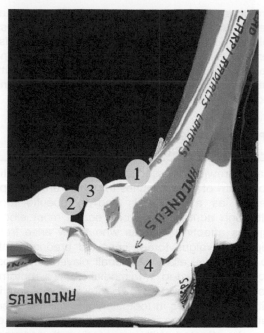

Fig. 3. A sawbones model of the lateral elbow, relevant muscular origins/insertions, and the lateral portals. (1) Proximal anterolateral portal; (2) anterolateral portal; (3) anterior radiocapitellar portal; (4) soft spot portal.

should be taken to protect the lateral ulnar collateral ligament (**Fig. 3**).[2] Techniques for protecting the lateral ulnar collateral ligament (LUCL) will be addressed in a later section.

Three portals are used posteriorly. The transtriceps/posteriocentral portal is located 3 cm proximal to the tip of the olecranon in the midline. This portal is useful for visualizing the posterior compartment, including the medial and lateral gutters. The proximal posterolateral portal is 2 to 3 cm proximal to the olecranon at the lateral border of the triceps tendon. Accessory posterolateral portals can be placed from the proximal posterolateral portal to the lateral soft spot; changing positions along this line facilitates entry to the posterolateral recess (**Fig. 4**).

Distorted anatomy is a relative contraindication to elbow arthroscopy.[3] Previous trauma, heterotopic ossification, or joint-deforming conditions such as osteoarthritis or rheumatoid arthritis merit extra caution to avoid inadvertent extraarticular placement of instruments and consequent nerve damage. Kelly and colleagues[1] noted joint contracture and rheumatoid arthritis to be the two most significant risk factors for postoperative complications such as nerve palsies.

The most common complication of elbow arthroscopy is prolonged drainage or superficial infection at portal sites. Lateral and posterolateral portals in particular are susceptible to developing

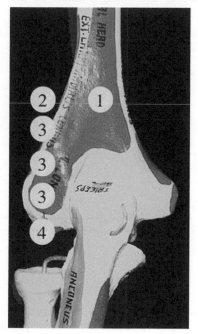

Fig. 4. A sawbones model of the posterior elbow, relevant muscular origins/insertions, and the posterior portals. (1) Posterocentral/transtricep portal; (2) proximal posterolateral portal; (3) accessory portals; (4) soft spot portal.

prolonged drainage postoperatively. The subcutaneous tissues at these sites are thinner and less reliable for sealing the space between the distended joint and the skin.[1] These complications can be avoided by careful, tight closure with multiple sutures. More serious complications include nerve injury or joint contracture.

SPORTS-RELATED INJURES
Anatomy and Biomechanics of Throwing

Hard throwing is associated with a characteristic spectrum of elbow injuries for which arthroscopy serves as a diagnostic and therapeutic tool. Although acute injuries can occur, most elbow injuries affecting athletes who throw arise from repetitive valgus forces imparted predominantly to the medial elbow. Baseball players are most commonly affected, with medial elbow symptoms accounting for up to 97% of elbow complaints in pitchers. Athletes in football, volleyball, lacrosse, tennis, gymnastics, and javelin throwing can likewise be affected. With increased youth participation in organized sports, it is not unusual that the age of onset is progressively earlier.[5]

An understanding of the anatomy and biomechanics of throwing is a necessary foundation to understanding the spectrum of pathophysiology unique to the throwing athlete. The baseball pitch is the most studied of the various overhead-throwing techniques, and is comprised of five stages (**Fig. 5**). In Stage 1, the windup, the elbow is flexed and the forearm pronated. In Stage 2, or early cocking, the ball leaves the nondominant hand as the shoulder begins to abduct and externally rotate. Stage 3, late cocking, begins when the forward foot contacts the ground. The shoulder abducts further and maximally rotates externally. The elbow is flexed between 90° and 120°, and the forearm pronates to 90°. In Stage 4, the shoulder musculature generates a rapid acceleration of the upper extremity, as much as $600,000°/s^2$. The humerus is internally rotated and abducted whereas the elbow is rapidly extended at up to $2500°/s^2$. Medial shear forces exceed 300 N, and lateral compressive forces exceed 900 N.[6] The tremendous kinetic energy of the throw is dissipated in Stage 5, the follow through, as the elbow reaches full extension. Deceleration occurs at $500,000°/s^2$ over 50 ms, exceeding the yield point of the MCL (33 N m).[5]

The primary restraint against the valgus force created during throwing is the MCL. The MCL is comprised of an anterior bundle, a posterior bundle, and a variable transverse bundle. The anterior bundle, believed to be the key stabilizer, originates from the inferior aspect of the medial epicondyle on the humerus and inserts onto the medial coronoid process, near the sublime tubercle. It is the strongest component of the

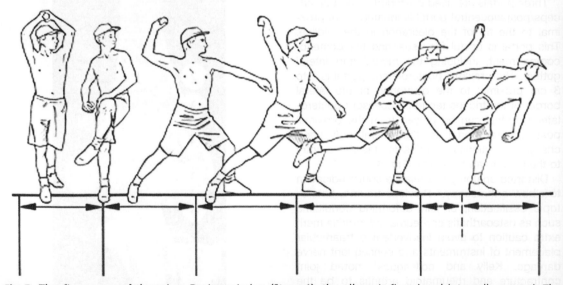

Fig. 5. The five stages of throwing. During windup (Stage 1), the elbow is flexed and internally rotated. The shoulder begins to abduct and externally rotate with early cocking (Stage 2), and reaches maximal external rotation during late cocking (Stage 3). The elbow is flexed and pronated at this stage, then rapidly extended during Stage 4, acceleration. The humerus is adducted and internally rotated. Energy is dissipated during follow through (Stage 5). (*Adapted from* Chen F, Rokito A, Jobe F. Medial elbow problems in the overhead-throwing athlete. JAAOS 2001;9:99–113; and DiGiovine NM, Jobe FW, Pink M, et al. An electromyographic analysis of the upper extremity in pitching. J Shoulder Elbow Surg 1992;1:15–25; with permission.)

MCL and remains eccentric to the axis of elbow motion, allowing it to function as the primary restraint to valgus force from 30° to 120° of elbow flexion. The anterior bundle is further divided into anterior and posterior bands. The anterior band is the primary restraint to valgus stress up to 90° of flexion, and becomes a secondary restrain with further flexion. The posterior band serves as a secondary restraint in lesser degrees of flexion, but becomes functionally more important between 60° and full flexion. The posterior band functions isometrically, and is functionally more important in the overhead athlete, as it is the primary restraint to valgus stress in higher degrees of flexion.[5] The posterior bundle of the MCL provides secondary stability to valgus stress when the elbow is flexed more than 90°. The posterior bundle is vulnerable to valgus stress only after the anterior bundle has been completely disrupted.[5] The transverse bundle, also referred to as Cooper's ligament, is a thickening of the caudal joint capsule, extending from the medial olecranon to the inferior medial coronoid process. It serves to expand the greater sigmoid notch, but offers little support against valgus stress. Muscular compression across the elbow functions synergistically with the wedge shape of the olecranon within the trochlea to provide additional varus-valgus stability.[6]

Pathophysiology of Medial Collateral Ligament Injury and Valgus Overload Syndrome

The repetitive valgus and extensor forces on the elbow during throwing cause attenuation and incompetence of the MCL. The resultant weakness and insufficiency of the stretched ligament increases the demand on the secondary stabilizers, including the ulnohumeral articulation, radiocapitellar articulation, the joint capsule, and the elbow musculature. Valgus overload is accentuated by a mechanically deficient MCL, leading to traction injuries to medial structures, as well as changes in the bony articulations of the lateral and posterior compartments.[7]

The differential diagnosis for medial elbow pain includes instability, ulnar neuritis, impingement, and capsular contracture. Symptoms of medial instability develop over time, and are reflective of the gradual attrition of the MCL as it is placed under chronic valgus stress. The moving valgus stress test, during which the elbow is brought through a range of motion while a valgus force is applied, is highly indicative of instability. A positive test results when a patient experiences pain between 70° and 120° of flexion. Nonoperative treatment of MCL instability consists of a 2- to 3-month rest period, followed by a graduated, pain-free throwing program that begins 3 months after return to normal strength. Using this regimen, 42% of athletes were returned to pre-injury level of play. Patients who fail conservative treatment, however, may be indicated for MCL reconstruction.[7]

Ulnar neuritis is another common condition that can present as medial elbow pain. The ulnar nerve is the most commonly injured neurovascular structure about the elbow, due in part to its anatomic features, and also to the characteristic muscle hypertrophy seen in throwers. During routine active flexion, the ulnar nerve experiences a three- to ninefold increase in pressure as it travels through the cubital tunnel. During the late cocking phase of throwing, in which the elbow is hyperflexed and the flexor carpi ulnaris (FCU) is contracted, compressive pressure within the cubital tunnel can increase as much as six- to twentyfold. In terms of its excursion, the nerve can translate as much as 7 mm anteromedially and lengthen as much as 4.7 mm during regular elbow flexion and extension.[8] However, this high degree of mobility can lead to subluxation or traction injury, particularly during the acceleration phase of throwing, when valgus forces are at the maximum. In a situation unique to throwing athletes, the ulnar nerve can be compressed proximally by a hypertrophied medial head of the triceps. Any of these pathologies can result in ulnar neuritis and symptoms of cubital tunnel syndrome. In a recent review, ulnar neuritis accounted for 15% of all upper extremity complaints in 72 professional baseball players.[9]

Patients with ulnar neuritis often complain of aching along the medial elbow or a feeling of heaviness to the arm. They also complain of paresthesias to the fourth and fifth digits, often worsening with throwing.[8] Suggestive findings of physical examination include a positive Tinel's sign and ulnar nerve subluxation on palpation of the flexed elbow. The elbow flexion test is a useful provocative maneuver in which symptoms are exacerbated with elbow hyperflexion and concomitant wrist extension. Ulnar neuritis is amenable to conservative treatment. In addition to avoiding throwing, a gentle course of physical therapy, icing, and antiinflammatory medication relieves most cases. A graduated throwing program can be restarted after 4 weeks of rest. If symptoms persist despite conservative treatment, a subcutaneous transposition can be performed to relieve pressure and traction on the nerve.[8] The senior author prefers to release all soft tissue constraints on the ulnar nerve (from the intermuscular septum to the fascia of the FCU) without transposing the nerve. The tissues are split on the posterior aspect, leaving the anterior tissues in place to prevent anterior subluxation of the nerve. The elbow is ranged after release to confirm that subluxation of the nerve is avoided. One advantage of not transposing the nerve is that future arthroscopy with a superomedial portal is feasible. In cases of ulnar neuritis with MCL instability, however, valgus laxity from an incompetent MCL must be addressed to prevent recurrence of symptoms. An MCL reconstruction should be undertaken when addressing the ulnar nerve pathology in throwers. Submuscular transposition is less favored, as it necessitates disruption of the flexor-pronator mass.[8]

MCL injury can lead to contact alterations in the posterior compartment.[10] Increased posteromedial shear forces, imparted by valgus stress, cause the olecranon to preferentially impinge against the medial wall of the olecranon fossa, predisposing to formation of osteophytes at this location. With the rapid extension in Stage 4 of throwing, impaction of the olecranon tip within the fossa occurs. As the articular tip of the olecranon impacts the posterior trochlea, a chondral defect, or kissing lesions, may develop on the humerus.[11] Osteophytes that develop at this articular tip of the olecranon are particularly prone to breakage and production of loose bodies,[6] which in turn may cause mechanical symptoms, such as blocking flexion or extension, or producing joint effusion and stiffness. In certain sports, such as boxing, repetitive hyperextension of the elbow can cause posterior compartment osteophytes and loose bodies in the absence of MCL injury.[12] With osteophytes and scar tissue impinging the elbow joint, the resultant reduction in range of motion can lead to capsular contracture. In these cases, the capsule must be released after joint debridement to allow full range of motion to be re-established.

As MCL integrity is compromised by repeated forceful throwing, a greater transfer of valgus stress is conveyed to the lateral compartment of the elbow, resulting in several lateral elbow pathologies. The increase in compressive and rotatory forces on the radiocapitellar articulation may lead to synovitis and chondromalacia. OCD and osteochondral fractures may in turn fragment and become loose bodies within the joint.[13] In skeletally immature athletes, valgus overload from excessive and overly forceful throwing can lead to capitellar OCD or Panner's disease, an avascular necrosis of the capitellum. Panner's disease is seen in children less than 10 years of age, presents as lateral elbow pain with restricted range of motion, and has a good prognosis if the offending activity is stopped. Capitellar OCD presents similarly to Panner's disease but occurs in adolescents. It is associated with loose body formation, and except in young patients with no radiographic changes, operative treatment leads to better outcomes. Any athlete with pathologic changes in the lateral elbow from excess compressive forces should be examined for MCL integrity.[11]

The differential diagnosis of lateral elbow pain in the athlete includes the consequences of valgus overload (OCD lesions, chondromalacia, loose bodies), lateral epicondylitis, and snapping plicae. Lateral epicondylitis is a common complaint in sports involving repetitive activities of the elbow, such as throwing a ball or swinging a golf club. There are several theories as to the cause of lateral epicondltitiis, with earlier literature attributing it to a chronic, degenerative tendinopathy featuring vascular proliferation and hyaline degeneration of the muscular origins of the extensor carpi radialis brevis (ECRB) and extensor digiti communis (EDC).[14,15] Others hypothesize of capsular involvement as well, suggesting a structural or anatomic predisposition. The radiocapitellar capsular complex (RCC) is an outcropping of capsule surrounding the radial head, separate from the annular ligament, and which can become inflamed and hypertrophied. Impingement of the RCC within the radiocapitellar joint results in lateral elbow pain.[16] Thickened plicae within the joint have also been implicated.[17,18] Plicae are capsulosynovial folds within the joint, remnants of embryologic septae, which can also become thickened and hardened when inflamed. Like the RCC, plicae caught within the radiocapitellar joint can impinge, causing pain and snapping.[19] Snapping usually occurs with flexion and extension, and is exacerbated by the repetitive movements of extension and pronation commonly seen in throwing or golfing.[17]

Clinically, tennis elbow presents as lateral elbow pain with resisted wrist extension or with grasping and lifting.[20–22] On physical examination, tenderness over the lateral epicondyle of the humerus and ECRB tendon origin can be consistently reproduced with palpation. If a snapping plicae is present, the patient's pain presents posterolaterally, and tenderness is elicited by palpating the posterolateral anconceus soft spot.[18] In addition, patients with plicae impinging between the capitellum and radial head may complain of snapping, catching, or locking on flexion-extension of the pronated forearm.[23,24] Reproducible and often palpable snapping that occurs over the anterior radial head as the fully flexed elbow is extended beyond 90° to 110° of flexion is diagnostic of plica syndromne.[17]

Lateral epicondylitis generally responds well to conservative therapy, and 80% to 90% of patients will have resolution of symptoms at 1 year with various combinations of rest, physical therapy, intraarticular steroids, and nonsteroidal anti-inflammatory drugs (NSAIDs). Patients with refractory lateral elbow pain are candidates for surgical treatment, which includes open and arthroscopic procedures.[3,15,22] The advantages of arthroscopy include limited skin incisions, preservation of muscle and tendon tissues overlying the ECRB and EDC origins, and the ability to treat concomitant intraarticular pathology.[20] Proponents also claim accelerated rehabilitation, earlier return to work/sports, and reduced morbidity.[21,25] Relative contraindications for arthroscopy in patients with lateral elbow pain include a concurrent diagnosis of posterolateral rotatory instability of the elbow or radial tunnel syndrome.[22]

THE ROLE OF ARTHROSCOPY IN MEDIAL ELBOW PAIN

Arthroscopy has emerged as an important tool in the diagnosis and treatment of throwing-related injuries. It allows for a thorough examination of intraarticular pathology in the elbow, as one series found preoperative radiographs to be only 27% sensitive for identification of loose bodies within the elbow.[11] Osteophyte and loose body debridement and contracture release are now typically performed arthroscopically.

The authors prefer arthroscopy in the supine or lazy lateral position, using an arm positioner to facilitate conversion to an open procedure, such as MCL reconstruction or ulnar nerve transposition

(**Fig. 1**). The authors examine and address the posterior compartment first. Often, osteophytes of the olecranon tip and olecranon are found to block extension (**Fig. 6**). This debridement is undertaken with transtriceps (viewing) and proximal posterolateral (working) portals. A distal posterolateral portal may be used for a retractor. The medial gutter, anterior ulnohumeral joint, lateral gutter, and radiocapitellar joint are then inspected. A dynamic valgus stress test, under direct visualization, is performed. In a normal elbow, a maximum of 1 to 2 mm opening is expected in the medial compartment with valgus stressing. Displacement greater than 2 mm is considered abnormal.[26] Arthroscopic evaluation of the MCL has become the gold standard in most institutions before an open reconstruction.[27] The radiocapitellar joint should be carefully inspected for osteochondral lesions and loose bodies through the anteromedial portal, the posterior radiocapitellar portal, or looking from a posterior portal with a 70° arthroscope (**Fig. 7**).

Capsular contracture can also be addressed arthroscopically. O'Driscoll recommends a stepwise release of contractures, beginning with synovectomy and removal of any soft tissue that may block motion due to bulk.[28] In the posttraumatic state, the elbow is expected to demonstrate pathology in most areas, consisting mostly of fibrotic tissue and synovitis. First, a proximal medial portal is created as a viewing portal. A lateral portal is established under direct visualization for use with instrumentation. Care is taken to start the anterior capsulotomy proximally to avoid the radial nerve, which travels intimately at the distal end of the capsule near the radial head

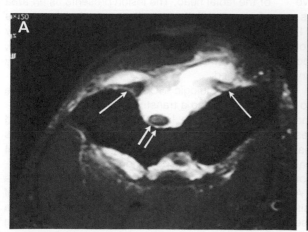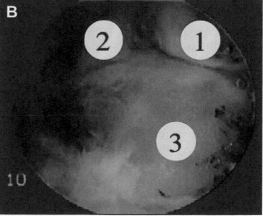

Fig. 6. The changes that occur in the posterior elbow secondary to overloading. (*A*) Axial MRI of distal humerus, demonstrating an effusion, humeral osteophytes (*single arrows*), and a loose body in olecranon fossa (*double arrow*). Up is posterior in this image. (*B*) Arthroscopic view of the medial elbow (left is medial, up is distal), demonstrating the tip of olecranon (**1**), posteromedial olecranon osteophyte (**2**), and the olecranon fossa (**3**).

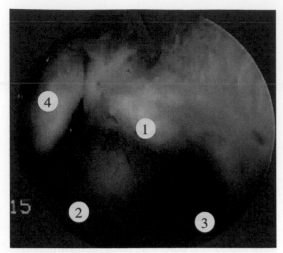

Fig. 7. A supracondylar ridge osteophyte (1) that can be present laterally. (2) Radial head; (3) coronoid fossa; (4) loose body.

and neck. If the shaver is used at this point, the suction should be shut off to prevent iatrogenic injury to the nerve.

After resection of the anterior capsule, straight posterior and posteriolateral portals are established for viewing and working, respectively, in the posterior compartment. Osteophytes are removed from the olecranon and coronoid process, to restore the normal contours of the olecranon fossa. The lateral gutter can be debrided through a lateral portal, and the chondral surfaces of the radial head and capitellum should be examined for defects.[29] The capsule is then released with a wide excision.[28] During debridement of the medial gutter and the excision of the posterior capsule, the ulnar nerve is most at risk for injury. Direct visualization of the ulnar nerve through an open incision is suggested if any question of its course behind the humerus exists. If preoperative flexion was limited (<100° arc of motion), the ulnar nerve should be decompressed or transposed to prevent traction injury postoperatively.[28]

Good results have been reported after arthroscopic treatment of elbow pathology in the throwing athlete. Studies examining outcomes after osteophyte debridement for posteromedial impingement, loose body removal, capsular release, treatment of OCD, and debridement for degenerative joint disease have been reported. A review of 187 elbow arthroscopies for diagnosis including posterior olecranon impingement, loose bodies, and degenerative disease, found a 92% good or excellent subjective satisfaction rate at an average follow-up of 42 months.[30] In this cohort, 47 of 55 professional baseball players

returned to their presurgical level of competition. Patients in this series who had undergone arthroscopic loose body removal reported more improved results compared with patients with degenerative joint disease. In young athletes who have undergone arthroscopic treatment of capitellar OCD or Panner's disease, short-term results are optimistic, with most patients returning to premorbid activity levels, including high-level throwing sports and gymnastics. Subjectively, patients report improved pain and increased range of motion.[13,31]

ARTHROSCOPIC TREATMENT OF LATERAL ELBOW PAIN

The arthroscopic technique for the surgical treatment of lateral epicondylitis has a few variations. With the patient's arm suspended from the lateral decubitus or supine position, the first step is a diagnostic arthroscopy of all compartments of the elbow. Direct visualization can be made of any snapping plicae or enflamed RCC that may be causing pain and mechanical symptoms. If these pathologies are present, the joint should be taken through passive range of motion exercises to observe for impingement.

Plicae are commonly visualized as large, enfolded synovial masses extending over the posterior aspect of the radial head, or as a tight shroud covering the anterior radial head with the elbow in flexion.[17] Plicae retract with supination, but tighten around the radial head with pronation, sometimes falling into the radiohumeral articulation (**Fig. 8**). The friction between the inflamed synovial fringe and the chondral surface may cause a characteristic kissing lesion adjacent to the articular margin of the radial head. The lesion presents as an area of chondral flattening with associated roughness and fibrillation (**Fig. 9**).[23] A local synovectomy and fringe excision of the plicae can be performed, although the kissing lesion itself is not directly addressed.

If a pathologic RCC is identified, it can be excised. Using a transtriceps or distal posterolateral portals, the lateral gutter is examined and a soft spot portal is established. This facilitates debridement of the posterior radiocapitellar joint and removal of the posterior RCC at its ulnar insertion. Excision of the posterior aspect releases the (often difficult to visualize) anterior part of the complex into the joint for easier access. The RCC is then debrided distally to normal-appearing annular ligament. Instruments should face away from the radial head to facilitate resection without damage to the articular surface. An anteromedial viewing portal, with an anterolateral working

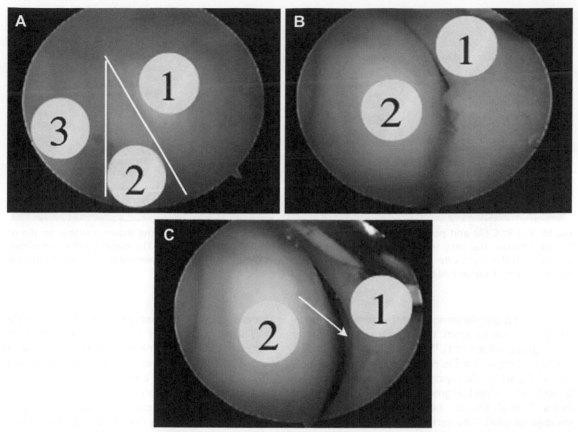

Fig. 8. Arthroscopic resection of a lateral plica. (*A*) The elbow is in flexion and radial head is almost completely covered. The white lines help delineate anatomic landmarks. (**1**) plica; (**2**) covered radial head; (**3**) capitellum. (*B*) With the elbow in extension, the radial head is uncovered. (**1**) plica; (**2**) unvocered radial head. (*C*) Debriding of plica reveals the rest of the radial head, neck, and annular ligament. (**1**) plica; (**2**) radial head; *arrow*, annular ligament deep to plica.

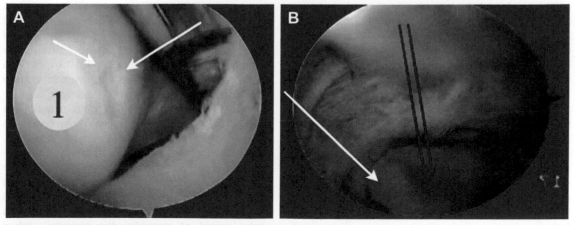

Fig. 9. Two examples of kissing lesions. (*A*) From the case in **Fig. 8**, the *arrow* points to the lesion. (**1**) radial head. The radiocapitellar joint is to the left and the radial neck to the right. (*B*) This is an example from a different case, with the *double black arrows* pointing to the kissing lesion. The *single white arrow* points to the radial head, the joint is to the right and the neck is to the left.

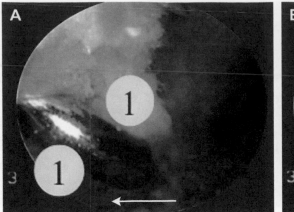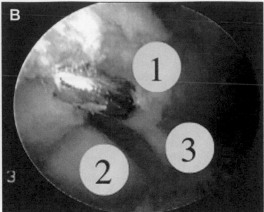

Fig. 10. Pre-RCC (*A*) and post-RCC (*B*) resection case. The pathologic RCC (**1**) with the shaver is sitting on the offending tissue. The only visible bony landmark is the capitellum (*white arrow*). The radial head is completely covered on the right side of the picture. The postresection (*B*) picture shows a resected RCC (**1**), capitellum (**2**), and uncovered radial head (**3**).

portal, will facilitate removal of the remaining anterolateral capsule from the equator of the radial head (**Figs. 10** and **11**).[16]

Degenerative lesions noted on the undersurface of the ECRB tendon grossly appear as discolored tissue with varying degrees of fibrous changes and tears,[21] and should be debrided as possible causes of pain. The tendon origins are debrided from the top of the capitellum to the midline of the radiocapitellar joint, with effort made to preserve normal appearing EDC tissue.[22] Debridement of the ECRB is considered complete when all visible pathologic tissue has been removed, and the overlying healthy EDC and extensor carpi radialis longus (ECRL) musculature can be seen.[25] If sclerotic bone is present, some advocate burring to bleeding bone, taking care to stay lateral and extraarticular. A lateral viewing portal or using a 70° arthroscope can assist in decortication.[32] An adequate anterolateral capsulectomy and debridement is performed when the radial head is exposed, without soft tissue impingement, with the elbow at 90° of flexion.

Capitellar OCD lesions are also amenable to arthroscopic treatment. Current surgical options include debridement, loose body excision, microfracture, chondral fixation, autologous bone graft, autologous osteochondral transplant, and autologous chondrocyte transplant. Most of these procedures involve an open approach, but arthroscopy is now playing a larger role. Using standard anteromedial, anterolateral, and posterolateral portals, full visualization and easy access to all involved joints can be established. Arthroscopy allows better visualization of not only the radiocapitellar joint but also the other joints of the elbow, allowing

for detection of accessory lesions (such as on the radial head, posterior capitellum, and trochlear notch of the capitellum) that may not be visible on conventional imaging or during an open approach (**Fig. 12**).[33] Lesions amenable to arthroscopic debridement have been found in the anterior capitellum, posteriolateral capitellum, and the posterior articular surface of the olecranon.[34] Loose bodies, reported in all compartments of the elbow, can be removed by arthroscopy.[31] Microfracturing through lateral portals has also been shown to be a viable treatment option, and if full range of motion is not obtained after debridement of lesions and loose bodies, arthroscopic capsulotomy may be performed.

The authors have successfully treated one patient with arthroscopic reduction and internal fixation of a loose cartilage piece. This procedure was supplemented with an autologous iliac crest bone graft. The patient presented with lateral elbow pain and was diagnosed by physical examination, radiography, and MRI (**Fig. 12**A, B). The patient's symptoms did not improve with activity modification and nonoperative treatment.

In the operating room (OR), the patient was placed in the supine position. The elbow was examined arthroscopically in a systematic fashion, from the posterior to medial to lateral compartments. No pathology was identified in the posterior or medial compartments. The distal posterolateral portal was used to visualize the capitellar lesion (**Fig. 12**C). After definition of the lesion and debridement of synovitis, the chondral defect was stabilized with a Freer elevator while a guide wire for a cannulated drill was introduced from the posterior humerus into the center of the lesion.

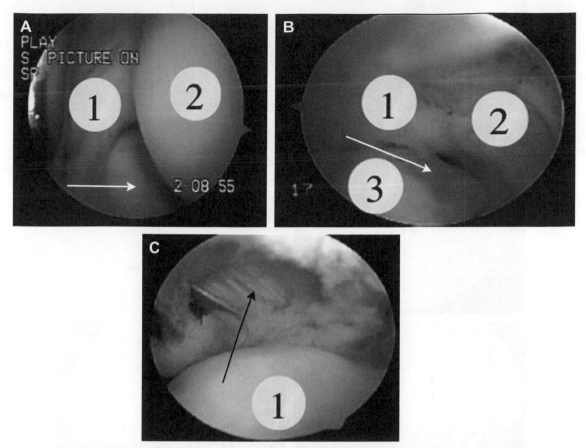

Fig.11. Pre-RCC (*A*) and post-RCC (*B, C*) resection. (*A*) The radial head is partially covered by RCC (**1**). The capitellum (**2**) and radial head (*arrow*) can be seen. (*B*) The lateral elbow after debridement; distal is left and the radiocapitellar joint is at 5 o'clock. The remnant RCC (**1**); capsule (**2**); and radial head (**3**) can be seen. A kissing lesion (*arrow*) is also visible. (*C*) The lateral elbow after debridement of capsule; left is distal. The radial head (**1**) and a grossly normal ECRB tendon (*arrow*) are shown.

A tunnel, for introduction of bone graft and suture placement, was created over the guide wire with the cannulated drill (**Fig. 12D**). The soft tissue guide for the drill was left in place while the drill and guide wire were removed. Two free ends of a polydioxanone suture (PDS) were passed through the guide and tunnel into the joint and retrieved with a grasper. Through the posterolateral portal, a 2.5-mm drill was used to create a bone tunnel proximomedial to the OCD lesion for passage of mattress sutures. An 18G spinal needle was used to introduce one end of a 25G steel wire segment into the joint (**Fig. 12E**). It was retrieved from the working portal, along with one end of the PDS. A loop was tied into the steel wire and the suture was placed into the loop. The wire loop was then cinched down onto the PDS, and used to guide the PDS back into the joint and out through the proximal drill hole to sit outside the arm (**Fig. 12F**). These steps were repeated for a PDS passed through

a proximolateral bone tunnel. Two more PDS ends were passed through the lesion into the joint. An 18G needle was introduced through the soft spot into the proximal radioulnar joint. Steel wire, as described above, was used to retrieve the PDS out through the soft spot. This step was repeated for a suture brought out the posterolateral capsule. The Freer elevator was used to tunnel under the soft tissue and retrieve all the sutures out the posterior wound. The suture pairs were then tied posteriorly to firmly fix the osteochondral fragment with multiple mattress sutures. Cancellous iliac crest bone graft was introduced into the lesion through the soft tissue drill guide. All wounds were closed with nylon sutures. The patient was splinted in 90° of flexion for approximately 5 days and then started on range of motion exercises. Follow-up at 3 months showed painless, full range of motion, and radiographic healing (**Fig. 12G, H**).

Preservation of the lateral collateral ligament (LCL) and LUCL is key to avoiding postoperative

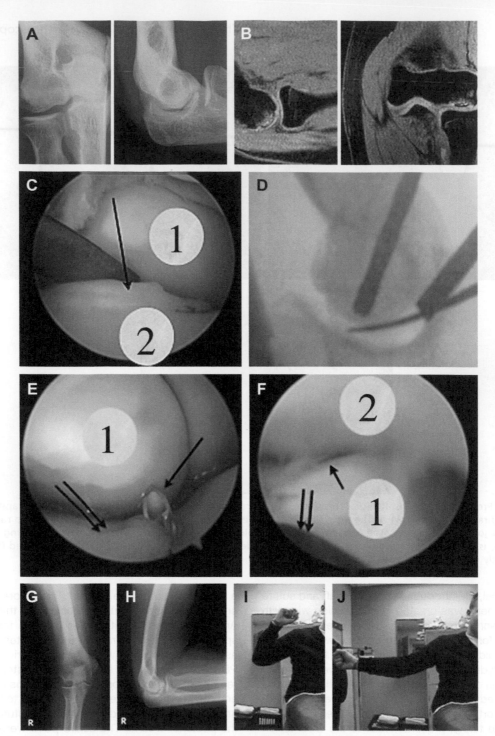

Fig. 12. Fixation and grafting of an OCD lesion. (*A*) The anterioposterior and lateral radiographs demonstrate capitellar lucency. (*B*) The sagittal and coronal T2 MR images demonstrate capitellar edema. (*C*) The loose lesion (*arrow*) on the capitellum (**2**) is being held in place by a Freer elevator. The radial head (**1**) can be seen. (*D*) The lateral miniflouro shot shows a proximal anteromedial cannulated drill in the capitellum; the Freer holds the reduction and the arthroscope enters the joint from the back. (*E*) An 18G needle, with 25G steel wire (*arrow*) is introduced through the anterocentral bone tunnel for mattress sutures. The radial head (**1**) and reduced OCD lesion (*double arrow*) are visible. (*F*) OCD lesion is being held in place with mattress sutures. A distal limb (*single arrow*) and the medial limb (*double arrow*) are visible, as are the medial capitellum (**1**) and radial head (**2**). (*G*) Three-month postoperative AP view of an OCD lesion. Although there is lucency within the capitellum, there is no collapse. (*H*) Lateral radiograph of the same elbow, demonstrating a preserved capitellum joint surface and a congruent joint. (*I*, *J*) Clinical picture of same elbow at 3 months. The patient's preoperative symptoms had resolved. The patient had painless, full range of motion.

instability.[20] In the technique described by Mullett and colleagues,[16] this was accomplished by limiting debridement to the equator of the radial head. A line bisecting the anterior half of the radial head was found to be an easily reproducible intra-articular anatomic landmark to demarcate the safe zone for resection of the extensor complex tendon origins. Debridement should not extend posterior to this line or anterior to the posterior one third of the radial head from the posterior approach. This preserves the radial collateral ligament and LUCL, which are necessary for maintaining joint stability.[14] Alternatively, resection to the limit of the visualization provided by the 30° arthroscope produces adequate release while protecting the LCLs, as does resecting to the border of the lateral intermuscular septum.[20,21] The joint can be filled with local anesthetic for postoperative pain relief.[20] There is no consensus on whether immediate active motion exercises or temporary immobilization with a splint (up to 14 days) following surgery is most beneficial.[16,20,21]

Arthroscopic excision of symptomatic plicae provides significant relief of pain and mechanical symptoms in most patients followed up to 12 or 13 months. Eleven of 12 athletes in one study were able to return to professional competition within an average of 4.8 months.[17–19,23] Results following arthroscopic release of the ECRB in patients with tennis elbow have been comparable to open debridement at 1- to 2-year follow-up, with both providing pain relief.[20–22,25] Arthroscopically treated patients did not demonstrate the increased morbidity, prolonged rehabilitation, and delayed return to work/sports associated with open techniques.[22] Most arthroscopically treated patients returned to work in 6 days to 3.2 weeks. In their series of 20 patients who underwent arthroscopic removal of a pathologic RCC, Mullett and colleagues[16] report patients returned to work in about 1 week, with relief from preoperative pain and return to preoperative sports level.

Fractures About the Elbow

Fracture care around the elbow is a new indication for elbow arthroscopy. The first case of arthroscopic fracture fixation in this part of the body was reported in 1997.[35] Sports-related capitellar, coronoid, and radial head fractures may be indications for arthroscopically assisted reduction and fixation.

Fractures of the Radial Head

Arthroscopic approaches have been described for open reduction, internal fixation of these fractures, and for radial head excision. Rolla and colleagues[36] described a technique for arthroscopic reduction with internal fixation (ARIF) of radial head fractures, which his group successfully used on patients with Mason 2, 3, and 4 fractures. An anteromedial viewing portal, with an anterolateral working portal, was first established for diagnostic and joint visualization purposes. Fracture reduction and fixation can then be undertaken from the lateral side. Visualization of the fracture is made from the posterolateral portal, whereas reduction with an elevator is performed through a lateral soft spot portal. Flexion of the elbow and supination of the forearm optimize the working field. Rolla and colleagues fixed their fractures with a single, cannulated screw, placed from an anterolateral portal and introduced at a 45° angle to the shaft. All aspects of the elbow joint were evaluated, and concomitant pathology (such as chondral lesions of the capitellum), were addressed. Their short-term results yielded no complications, and all patients returned to premorbid activity within 6 months.[36]

If the head is left in suit (after either nonoperative treatment or internal fixation), symptomatic, post-traumatic arthritis is a commonly encountered sequaelae. Operative treatment choices of this complication are radial head excision or replacement. When contemplating radial head resection, there is considerable debate in the literature as to the timing of resection.[37,38] The results of delayed, open resection are mixed, but late arthroscopic radial head resection may offer an alternative treatment.[39–41] The authors believe, however, that isolated radial head resection is rarely, if ever, indicated in an active individual because this can exacerbate instability, resulting in premature arthrosis.

Another common sequelae of radial head fractures, regardless of initial treatment modality, is elbow stiffness.[29,42] Arthroscopic capsular release for stiffness secondary to other traumatic injuries has been described in the past.[43,44] It has also been used successfully for arthrofibrosis following nondisplaced radial head fractures that were treated nonoperatively.[29]

Fractures of the Capitellum

Capitellar fractures can be complex injuries, with a high complication rate including malunion, nonunion, loss of fixation, and stiffness.[45] Adequate visualization, particularly of an anterior coronal shear-type injury, is difficult even through an extended open approach and in these cases, arthroscopy may be helpful. Three types of capitellar fractures have been described. Type 1 fractures, also known as Hans Steinthal fractures, are shear fractures of the capitellum in the coronal plane. They usually involve a significant part of the osseous capitellum and a portion of the lateral trochlea. Type 2 fractures, known as Kocher Lorenz fractures, are osteochondral avulsions of the articular surface of the capitellum. Type 3 fractures involve comminution of the capitellum.

Whereas reducible type 1 fractures may be treated nonoperatively, most capitellar fractures are treated with open reduction, internal fixation (unreduced type 1), or capitellar excision (types 2 and 3 fractures). Open treatment is traditionally described through a lateral Kocher approach. As discussed above, the neurovascular structures (in particular the posterior interosseous nerve) and LUCL are most at risk in this approach.[46] An arthroscopic approach to these fractures minimizes risk to the lateral ligaments, allows better visualization of all joint spaces of the elbow, and facilitates earlier rehabilitation.

Capitellar fractures characteristically displace proximally (**Fig. 13**A, B). ARIF of a capitellum fracture begins with reduction of the proximally displaced fragment. A proximal anterolateral portal is established under fluoroscopic control to allow for insertion of a trochar proximal to the fragment, which is then reduced by extending the elbow and, if necessary, pushing the fragment distally with the trochar. The elbow is flexed more than 90° so that the radial head will lock the capitellum into position. If flexing the elbow displaces the fragment, then the trocar, or a Freer elevator, is inserted like a shoehorn into the radiocapitellar joint to keep the fragment in place as the radial head glides over the capitellum and the elbow is fully flexed (**Fig. 13**C). Displaced type 2 fractures are more challenging. The reduction maneuver may be similar, or may require retrieval and distal traction on the fragment with a small skin hook through the posterior radiocapitellar portal. Proximal

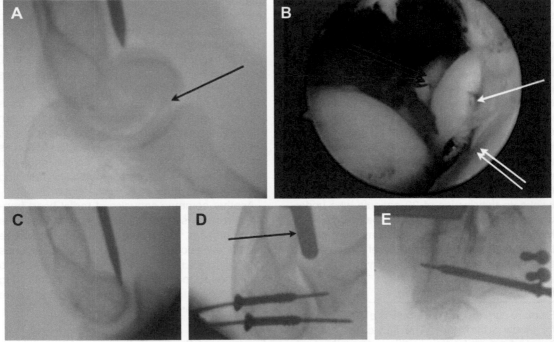

Fig. 13. Arthroscopic fixation of a capitellar fracture. The unreduced fracture can be seen indirectly (*A*) and directly (*B*). (*A*) A lateral fluoroscopic image of an extended elbow prereduction. The black arrow points to articular stepoff at the fracture line, with the arthroscopic trocar in the supracapitellar fossa, ready to assist with reduction. (*B*) The arthroscopic view, from proximal with a 70° scope, of the extended, lateral elbow. From proximal to distal, landmarks include the humerus (*double white arrow*), the fracture line with a displaced capitellar segment (*single white arrow*), and the radial head (*double black arrow*). Lateral fluoroscopic images demonstrate fracture reduction with elbow flexion and an elevator (*C*); and fracture fixation with two proximal anteromedial cannulated screws (*D*). The black arrow highlights the position of the 70° scope, coming over the top through the proximal anterolateral portal. (*E*) The AP fluoro shot demonstrates the final fixation with two proximal anteromedial, and one lateral to medial, cannulated screws. The lateral screw was used as a blocking screw to prevent proximal migration of the reduction screws.

anteromedial and posterior portals are used to visualize and debride the fracture. An accessory posterior radiocapitellar portal may be necessary. There is frequently some comminution or plastic deformation of the distal humerus that prevents an anatomic reduction and these bone fragments must be debrided from the posterior radiocapitellar portal.

For type 1 fractures, guide wires for cannulated 3.5 or 4.5 screws are then placed under fluoroscopic guidance (**Fig. 13**D). The position and length of the screws can be confirmed by direct arthroscopic inspection. After measuring the requisite length of the screws, the wires are advanced, to prevent inadvertent pullout, and the holes are drilled and the screws inserted. A lateral-to-medial blocking screw can be placed just proximal to the capitellum to prevent proximal migration of the proximal anteromedial screws (**Fig. 13**E). For reducible type 2 fractures, the osseous fragment is usually too thin to accept a screw and must be fixed with transosseous sutures (see the transosseous fixation of an OCD lesion for the technique). Postoperative management should consist of early range of motion to prevent stiffness.[47] If the fixation is felt to be tenuous, healing should be prioritized over motion, and the joint should be immobilized until fracture healing is evident. Joint motion can then be reliably restored with subsequent arthroscopic capsulectomy and contracture release.

For unreducible type 2 and type 3 capitellar fractures, excision of the chondral fragments is the treatment of choice. This procedure can be approached through a lateral open incision or arthroscopically, which offers the dual advantages of minimized risk of nerve and ligamentous damage and allowing full examination of all elbow compartments. Standard anteromedial (viewing) and anterolateral (working) portals can be used.[35] After hematoma evacuation and lavage, the fracture fragments are identified. If the fragments are too small for fixation, they can be debrided as loose bodies. Other joint surfaces, in particular the radial head, should be inspected for traumatic defects. Early range of motion exercises are advocated postoperatively to prevent arthrofibrosis.

Fractures of the Coronoid

The coronoid has been established as an important stabilizer for the elbow, especially against varus and rotatory stress. This anterior process of the olecranon is usually fractured in association with an elbow subluxation or dislocation. Until recently, all operative treatment of coronoid fractures was performed through an open approach, requiring either an extensive straight posterior approach, or a combined medial and lateral approach.[36] Both methods necessitated extensive soft tissue dissection, including potential capsular release to achieve adequate visualization.[48]

Arthroscopic treatments of varying coronoid fracture sizes have now been documented.[49,50] This technique may allow fixation of coronoid fractures, with less insult to the soft tissue, particularly the anterior capsule. Arthroscopy can also be used to assist and minimize a more formal open reduction, internal fixation of complex coronoid fractures.

A standard elbow arthroscopy setup is used according to the surgeon's preference. An anteromedial viewing portal is established, followed by 1 to 2 anterolateral portals for instruments and retractors.[48] After sufficient lavage and debridement, the coronoid fracture is assessed, reduction attempted, and size appropriate fixation is used. Adams and colleagues[51] advocate debrided and excision of small tip fractures; it is the senior author's preference to excise only those bony fragments without soft tissue attachments.

Reduction techniques include using arthroscopic graspers or ring curettes placed through the anterolateral portal, or an over the top ACL guide placed in the medial portal. The arthroscope provides viewing from a lateral portal. After confirmation of reduction, a posterior to anterior guide wire is inserted. A second guide wire may be helpful for derotational purposes when necessary.

Screw fixation can be reinforced with arthroscopic suture fixation. A mattress suture is passed through the anterior capsule, near its insertion on to the coronoid, using an arthroscopic suture passing system (ie, Spectrum System, Linvatec Corp, Largo, Florida). Through a small incision on the dorsal ulna, a Freer elevator is then used to dissect the soft tissue off the medial ulna, with care taken to stay deep to the ulnar nerve. A Hewson suture passer is used to retrieve one end of the suture. Laterally, an 18G needle is introduced through the soft spot into the proximal radioulnar joint. Following arthroscopic confirmation of placement, a Hewson suture passer, or equivalent, is used to retrieve the lateral limb of the suture, which is then passed subcutaneously into the dorsal incision.[48]

Arthroscopy does not preclude open surgery. If an adequate reduction and fixation cannot be obtained arthroscopically, a limited open incision can be made for plate fixation. After fixation, reduction and stability are evaluated arthroscopically and fluoroscopically. Any additional ligamentous repair can be performed in a traditional open technique or with an arthroscopic imbrication.[51] Postoperative instructions should include early range of motion exercises to avoid stiffness. Between the two published series, all patients achieved a stable elbow with a functional range of motion. There was one case of asymptomatic heterotopic ossification, one residual instability (which resolved after a secondary procedure), and one ulnar nerve neuropathy (which resolved after an ulnar nerve transposition).[51]

Elbow arthroscopy is uniquely suited to treat injuries in athletes, whether they are chronic overuse types or fractures about the elbow joint. Given the numerous neurovascular structures about the elbow, a thorough understanding of anatomy is critical for performing elbow arthroscopy and any doubt on the course of nerves, such as following an ulnar nerve transposition, should prompt consideration for an open procedure. In patients with pain stemming from osteophytes, loose bodies, or hypertrophied soft tissue, such as plicae or a pathologic RCC, elbow arthroscopy offers a quick, reliable, and effective treatment. In patients requiring more complex procedures, such as MCL reconstruction or fracture fixation, elbow arthroscopy can be a useful adjunctive tool to fully visualize the joint, to confirm a diagnosis, or to evaluate a reduction. The role of elbow arthroscopy in fracture care is nascent, but as surgeons develop technical expertise in arthroscopy and indications for minimally invasive procedures increase, it will likely become a powerful and indispensable tool for the orthopedic surgeon.

REFERENCES

1. Kelly EW, Morrey BF, O'Driscoll SW. Complications of elbow arthroscopy. J Bone Joint Surg Am 2001; 83(1):25–34.

2. Abboud JA, Ricchetti ET, Tjoumakaris F, et al. Elbow arthroscopy: basic setup and portal placement. J Am Acad Orthop Surg 2006;14(5):312–8.

3. Dodson CC, Nho SJ, Williams RJ 3rd, et al. Elbow arthroscopy. J Am Acad Orthop Surg 2008;16(10): 574–85.

4. Savoie FH 3rd. Guidelines to becoming an expert elbow arthroscopist. Arthroscopy 2007;23(11): 1237–40.

5. Chen FS, Rokito AS, Jobe FW. Medial elbow problems in the overhead-throwing athlete. J Am Acad Orthop Surg 2001;9(2):99–113.

6. Safran M, Ahmad CS, Elattrache NS. Ulnar collateral ligament of the elbow. Arthroscopy 2005;21(11): 1381–95.

7. Grace SP, Field LD. Chronic medial elbow instability. Orthop Clin North Am 2008;39(2):213–9, vi.

8. Keefe DT, Lintner DM. Nerve injuries in the throwing elbow. Clin Sports Med 2004;23(4):723–42, xi.

9. Andrews JR, Timmerman LA. Outcome of elbow surgery in professional baseball players. Am J Sports Med 1995;23(4):407–13.

10. Ahmad CS, Park MC, Elattrache NS. Elbow medial ulnar collateral ligament insufficiency alters posteromedial olecranon contact. Am J Sports Med 2004; 32(7):1607–12.

11. Cain EL Jr, Dugas JR, Wolf RS, et al. Elbow injuries in throwing athletes: a current concepts review. Am J Sports Med 2003;31(4):621–35.

12. Valkering KP, van der Hoeven H, Pijnenburg BC. Posterolateral elbow impingement in professional boxers. Am J Sports Med 2008;36(2):328–32.

13. Takahara M, Mura N, Sasaki J, et al. Classification, treatment, and outcome of osteochondritis dissecans of the humeral capitellum. J Bone Joint Surg Am 2007;89(6):1205–14.

14. Smith AM, Castle JA, Ruch DS. Arthroscopic resection of the common extensor origin: anatomic considerations. J Shoulder Elbow Surg 2003;12(4):375–9.

15. Brooks-Hill AL, Regan WD. Extra-articular arthroscopic lateral elbow release. Arthroscopy 2008; 24(4):483–5.

16. Mullett H, Sprague M, Brown G, et al. Arthroscopic treatment of lateral epicondylitis: clinical and cadaveric studies. Clin Orthop Relat Res 2005;439:123–8.

17. Antuna SA, O'Driscoll SW. Snapping plicae associated with radiocapitellar chondromalacia. Arthroscopy 2001;17(5):491–5.

18. Kim DH, Gambardella RA, Elattrache NS, et al. Arthroscopic treatment of posterolateral elbow impingement from lateral synovial plicae in throwing athletes and golfers. Am J Sports Med 2006;34(3): 438–44.

19. Ruch DS, Papadonikolakis A, Campolattaro RM. The posterolateral plica: a cause of refractory lateral elbow pain. J Shoulder Elbow Surg 2006;15(3): 367–70.

20. Jerosch J, Schunck J. Arthroscopic treatment of lateral epicondylitis: indication, technique and early results. Knee Surg Sports Traumatol Arthrosc 2006; 14(4):379–82.

21. Owens BD, Murphy KP, Kuklo TR. Arthroscopic release for lateral epicondylitis. Arthroscopy 2001; 17(6):582–7.

22. Kalainov DM, Makowiec RL, Cohen MS. Arthroscopic tennis elbow release. Tech Hand Up Extrem Surg 2007;11(1):2–7.

23. Clarke RP. Symptomatic, lateral synovial fringe (plica) of the elbow joint. Arthroscopy 1988;4(2): 112–6.

24. Akagi M, Nakamura T. Snapping elbow caused by the synovial fold in the radiohumeral joint. J Shoulder Elbow Surg 1998;7(4):427–9.

25. Baker CL Jr, Baker CL 3rd. Long-term follow-up of arthroscopic treatment of lateral epicondylitis. Am J Sports Med 2008;36(2):254–60.

26. Field LD, Altchek DW. Evaluation of the arthroscopic valgus instability test of the elbow. Am J Sports Med 1996;24(2):177–81.

27. O'Holleran JD, Altchek DW. The thrower's elbow: arthroscopic treatment of valgus extension overload syndrome. HSS J 2006;2(1):83–93.

28. O'Driscoll SW. Arthroscopic treatment for osteoarthritis of the elbow. Orthop Clin North Am 1995; 26(4):691–706.

29. Lapner PC, Leith JM, Regan WD. Arthroscopic debridement of the elbow for arthrofibrosis resulting from nondisplaced fracture of the radial head. Arthroscopy 2005;21(12):1492.

30. Reddy AS, Kvitne RS, Yocum LA, et al. Arthroscopy of the elbow: a long-term clinical review. Arthroscopy 2000;16(6):588–94.

31. Krijnen MR, Lim L, Willems WJ. Arthroscopic treatment of osteochondritis dissecans of the capitellum: report of 5 female athletes. Arthroscopy 2003;19(2): 210–4.

32. Baker CL Jr, Murphy KP, Gottlob CA, et al. Arthroscopic classification and treatment of lateral epicondylitis: two-year clinical results. J Shoulder Elbow Surg 2000;9(6):475–82.

33. Robla J, Hechtman KS, Uribe JW, et al. Chondromalacia of the trochlear notch in athletes who throw. J Shoulder Elbow Surg 1996;5(1):69–72.

34. Bojanic I, Ivkovic A, Boric I. Arthroscopy and microfracture technique in the treatment of osteochondritis dissecans of the humeral capitellum: report of three adolescent gymnasts. Knee Surg Sports Traumatol Arthrosc 2006;14(5):491–6.

35. Feldman MD. Arthroscopic excision of type II capitellar fractures. Arthroscopy 1997;13(6):743–8.

36. Rolla PR, Surace MF, Bini A, et al. Arthroscopic treatment of fractures of the radial head. Arthroscopy 2006;22(2):233.e1–6.

37. Wallenbock E, Potsch F. Resection of the radial head: an alternative to use of a prosthesis? J Trauma 1997;43(6):959–61.

38. Janssen RP, Vegter J. Resection of the radial head after Mason type-III fractures of the elbow: follow-up at 16 to 30 years. J Bone Joint Surg Br 1998;80(2):231–3.

39. Broberg MA, Morrey BF. Results of delayed excision of the radial head after fracture. J Bone Joint Surg Am 1986;68(5):669–74.

40. Stephen IB. Excision of the radial head for closed fracture. Acta Orthop Scand 1981;52(4):409–12.

41. Menth-Chiari WA, Poehling GG, Ruch DS. Arthroscopic resection of the radial head. Arthroscopy 1999;15(2):226–30.

42. Radin EL, Riseborough EJ. Fractures of the radial head. A review of eighty-eight cases and analysis of the indications for excision of the radial head and non-operative treatment. J Bone Joint Surg Am 1966;48(6):1055–64.

43. Kim SJ, Kim HK, Lee JW. Arthroscopy for limitation of motion of the elbow. Arthroscopy 1995;11(6):680–3.

44. Timmerman LA, Andrews JR. Arthroscopic treatment of posttraumatic elbow pain and stiffness. Am J Sports Med 1994;22(2):230–5.

45. Tsuji H, Wada T, Oda T, et al. Arthroscopic, macroscopic, and microscopic anatomy of the synovial fold of the elbow joint in correlation with the common extensor origin. Arthroscopy 2008;24(1):34–8.

46. Dushuttle RP, Coyle MP, Zawadsky JP, et al. Fractures of the capitellum. J Trauma 1985;25(4):317–21.

47. Hardy P, Menguy F, Guillot S. Arthroscopic treatment of capitellum fracture of the humerus. Arthroscopy 2002;18(4):422–6.

48. Hausman MR, Klug RA, Qureshi S, et al. Arthroscopically assisted coronoid fracture fixation: a preliminary report. Clin Orthop Relat Res 2008; 466(12):3147–52.

49. Regan W, Morrey B. Fractures of the coronoid process of the ulna. J Bone Joint Surg Am 1989; 71(9):1348–54.

50. O'Driscoll SW, Morrey BF, Korinek S, et al. Elbow subluxation and dislocation. A spectrum of instability. Clin Orthop Relat Res 1992;280:186–97.

51. Adams JE, Merten SM, Steinmann SP. Arthroscopic-assisted treatment of coronoid fractures. Arthroscopy 2007;23(10):1060–5.

Arthroscopic and Open Radial Ulnohumeral Ligament Reconstruction for Posterolateral Rotatory Instability of the Elbow

Felix H. Savoie III, MD[a,b,*], Larry D. Field, MD[c], Daniel J. Gurley, MD[d]

KEYWORDS

- Elbow • Radial ulnohumeral ligament
- Arthroscopic radial ulnohumeral ligament reconstruction
- Open radial ulnohumeral ligament reconstruction
- Posterolateral rotatory instability

Interest in the diagnosis and treatment of postero-lateral rotatory instability (PLRI) of the elbow has grown since the original description by O'Driscoll and colleagues in 1991. PLRI has been described as an instability pattern of the elbow that results from an incompetent radial ulnohumeral ligament complex (RULC).[1] Anatomic studies have attempted to define the involved tissue. Dunning and colleagues,[2] stated that the radial ulnohumeral ligament (RUHL) and the radial collateral ligament (RCL) must be sectioned to achieve PLRI. They also stated that they could not visually differentiate the two ligaments at their humeral origin. They could only differentiate the RUHL from the RCL by identifying the distal extent of the RUHL at the supinator crest of the ulna.[2] Seki and colleagues[3] were able to show that sectioning just the anterior band of the lateral collateral complex induced instability. This suggests that an intact RUHL cannot stabilize the elbow. These data demonstrate that the entity of PLRI is a spectrum of injury.

Although originally described as sequelae of an elbow dislocation, these anatomic studies and a later report by Kalainov and Cohen support the authors' experience that there is a continuum of injury between PLRI and frank elbow dislocation.[1,4,5]

This instability is best demonstrated clinically with the pivot shift test of the elbow. This test, as first described by O'Driscoll and colleagues,[1] performed with the patient in the supine position, may elicit gross instability or simply pain and apprehension. There are 2 other clinical tests described by Regan and Lapner[6] that include (1) pain when pushing up from an armchair with the palms facing inward and (2) having the patient push up from a prone or wall-leaning position first, with the forearms maximally pronated, and then repeating the test with the forearms supinated, reproducing either pain or instability, or both.[7]

The authors prefer to examine the elbow with the patient in the prone position and to use the

a Department of Orthopaedics, Tulane University School of Medicine, 1430 Tulane Avenue SL-32, New Orleans, LA 70112, USA
b Tulane Institute of Sports Medicine, New Orleans, LA 70118, USA
c Shoulder and Elbow Service, Mississippi Sports Medicine and Orthopaedic Center, Jackson, MS 39202, USA
d College Park Family Care Center, Overland Park, KS 66212, USA
* Corresponding author. Department of Orthopaedics, Tulane University School of Medicine, 1430 Tulane Avenue SL-32, New Orleans, LA 70112.
E-mail address: busavoie@aol.com (F.H. Savoie III).

Hand Clin 25 (2009) 323–329
doi:10.1016/j.hcl.2009.05.010

table as a base to stabilize the humerus. Examination of the elbow in this position mimics the examination of a flexed knee, and the findings seem to be more easily reproduced between examiners. Examination begins by manually trying to rotate the forearm from the humerus in 90° of flexion, palpating the radiocapitellar joint, and using the wrist to supinate and rotate the forearm to reproduce the radial column subluxation away from the humerus. The radial head movement on the capitellum is more easily seen and felt in this position, and the elbow can be flexed and extended while maintaining the subluxation force.

Imaging studies for PLRI can be helpful. Radiographs may reveal an avulsion fragment from the posterior humeral lateral epicondyle in acute cases. However, often radiographs are normal. A stress radiograph or fluoroscopy while performing the pivot shift test may show the radial head and proximal ulna moving together in a subluxated and posterolaterally rotated position. MRI of the elbow has been described to identify a lesion in the RUHL.[8] The authors find that MRIs are most helpful when contrast is added. This can be either a formal arthrogram or, in the case of office MRI, an injection of 20 to 30 mL of sterile normal saline just before the scan can greatly enhance the effectiveness of the test.

Although much has been written about the pathoanatomy and biomechanics of the lesion, little has been reported on the surgical treatment of these patients. There are no large published series on the outcomes of the surgical treatment of PLRI. This study reviews the outcomes of the authors' experiences with arthroscopic repair, plication, and open grafting techniques previously described by Savoie and other colleagues.[4]

SURGICAL TECHNIQUE

Most cases of simple dislocation respond to nonoperative management. In cases in which the instability recurs, or in which acute evaluation reveals a significant tear or avulsion, surgical treatment may be indicated. Arthroscopy of the acutely injured elbow demands speed and precision. A concrete preoperative plan must be formulated and followed, with adjustment made for arthroscopic findings. Patients with significant coronoid fracture, associated radial head fracture, or distal humerus fracture are not included in this report.

ARTHROSCOPIC REPAIR

In the elbow with an acute or chronic avulsion of the RULC, arthroscopic repair can be effective. The procedure begins with the establishment of a proximal anterior medial portal and a diagnostic anterior compartment arthroscopy. In the acute setting, it may be necessary to establish a lateral portal to clean out the associated hematoma (**Fig. 1**). The tearing of the anterior capsule is readily apparent. In acute dislocations, one can often also see the damage to the brachialis muscle through the torn capsule (**Figs. 2**A, B). The main area of interest here is to view the annular ligament for damage and place a suture in it if necessary. One can also view "around the corner" of the proximal capitellum for damage to the collateral ligament part of the RULC. The arthroscope is then placed into the posterior central portal, and the hematoma in the back of the elbow compartment is evacuated by way of a proximal posterior lateral portal. Both of these portals need to be relatively proximal to allow for the later repair of the ligament, usually at least 3 cm above the colcannon tip. A view of the medial gutter will show hemorrhage, and sometimes tearing of the capsule, near the posterior aspect of the medial epicondyle (**Fig. 3**). The lateral gutter and capsule is then evaluated. It is very important to stay close to the ulna as the lateral gutter is evaluated and the hematoma debrided, as the avulsed ligament and bone fragments are displaced distally and may inadvertently be removed by the shaver (**Fig. 4**). The lateral aspect of the posterior humerus should also be lightly debrided and the site of avulsion localized. It is usually directly lateral and slightly inferior to the center of the olecranon fossa. Once the area of damage has been defined, an arthroscopic anchor may be placed into the humerus at the site of origin of the RUHL (**Fig. 5**). The limbs of the suture are then retrieved to place two horizontal mattress sutures through the noninjured part of the ligament. In the case of a bony

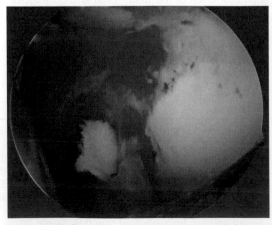

Fig. 1. A view from the proximal anterior medial portal of the hematoma, often seen in an acute dislocation.

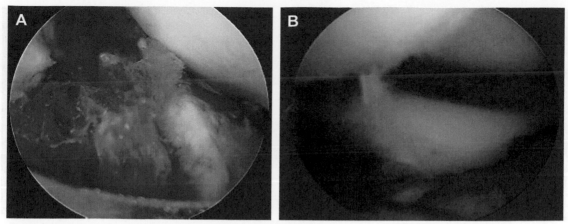

Fig. 2. (*A*) The arthroscopic view of the damaged brachialis and torn anterior capsule often noted in acute dislocations. (*B*) The laxity seen in the annular ligament and the displacement of the radial head from the capitellum in acute and chronic PLRI is visualized from the medial portal.

avulsion, one set of sutures is placed around the bone fragment and, the other, distal to the fragment (**Fig. 6**). The sutures are tensioned while the physician is viewing the lesion with the arthroscope, which should have the effect of pushing it (the arthroscope) out of the lateral gutter. The patient's elbow is then extended, and the sutures are tied beneath the anconeus muscle, tightening the ligament. Motion and stability are then evaluated with the arthroscope back in the anterior compartment (**Fig. 7**).

ARTHROSCOPIC PLICATION

The development of an arthroscopic technique for the treatment of chronic PLRI was described by Smith and colleagues[4] in 2001. Chronic

posterolateral instability is more readily seen during examination under anesthesia and on arthroscopic evaluation. While the examiner is viewing from the proximal anterior medial portal, the ulna and radial head can be seen to subluxate posterolaterally during the performance of a pivot shift test. In most cases, the annular ligament is intact, as the entire proximal radioulnar joint shifts on the humerus. One common finding is the ability to move an arthroscope placed down the posterolateral gutter from the posterior central portal straight across the ulnohumeral articulation into the medial gutter. This maneuver is not possible in a stable elbow and is termed the "drive-through sign" of the elbow. It is somewhat analogous to the "drive-through" sign in shoulder instability (**Fig. 8**). The elimination of the laxity that allows this maneuver is one of the key aspects of

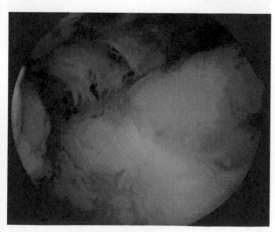

Fig. 3. The concomitant tearing of the capsule of the medial capsule in acute instability is visualized from a posterior portal.

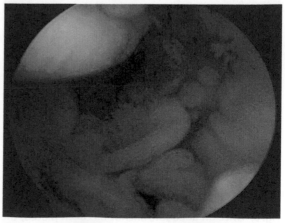

Fig. 4. The bone and soft tissue fragments often seen in the lateral gutter in acute dislocation.

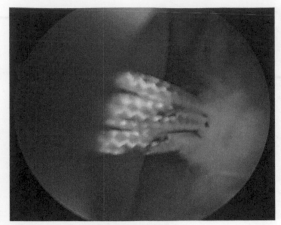

Fig. 5. The site of anchor placement into the humerus just lateral to the olecranon fossa of the humerus as viewed from the posterior portal.

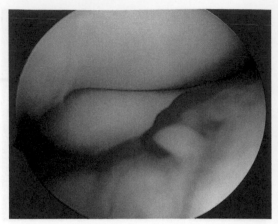

Fig. 7. The repaired ligament is visualized from the posterior portal.

confirming an adequate arthroscopic reconstruction in patients with PLRI.

The arthroscopic technique for chronic instability has two key features: plication of the two major components of the complex and repair of the complex to the humerus. Both components can be managed by arthroscopic techniques if there is enough ligamentous and capsular tissue. This assessment is in part determined by the preoperative evaluation, including palpation of the structures in the area to be reconstructed, the amount of previous surgery, and the tissue present on MR arthrogram findings. If adequate tissue is present, the tissue in the posterolateral gutter is assessed arthroscopically and prepared with a shaver or rasp. About four to seven absorbable sutures are then placed in oblique fashion

beginning at the most distal extent of the RUHL complex attachment to the ulna. The sutures are placed into the lateral gutter by an 18-gauge spinal needle that slides along the radial border of the ulna. The first suture is delivered into the joint through the midportion of the annular ligament (**Fig. 9**A). Subsequent sutures are brought into the joint in a progressively more proximal position. Each suture is immediately retrieved with a retrograde suture retriever that passes into the joint from the posterior lateral aspect of the lateral epicondyle (see **Fig. 9**B). It is important that the retrograde retriever comes under the entire RUHL near its proximal attachment to the humerus. Once all the sutures have been placed, they are retrieved one at a time percutaneously through the existing skin portals under, or in some cases over, the anconeus muscle; the sutures are pulled to create

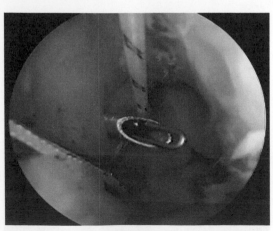

Fig. 6. Once an adequate anchor has been placed, the sutures are retrieved through the torn radioulnohumeral ligament in preparation for repair.

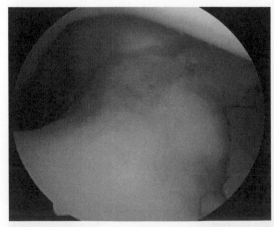

Fig. 8. The "drive-through sign" of the elbow is performed by placing the arthroscope into the lateral gutter and moving it straight across the ulnohumeral articulation into the medial gutter.

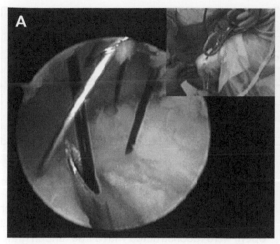
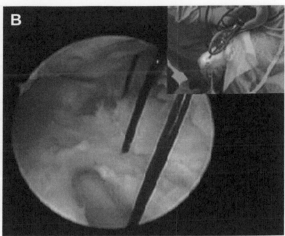

Fig. 9. (*A*) The suture is retrieved using a retrograde retriever introduced along the posterior aspect of the lateral epicondyle and under the proximal end of the RUHL complex. (*B*) The views of the closed radial gutter when all the sutures are placed and just before the sutures are tensioned.

tension and to evaluate the plication. If the reconstruction has been properly performed, and the tissue is adequate for plication, the arthroscope is driven out of the lateral gutter as this tensioning occurs. The arthroscope is then removed, the elbow is extended, and the sutures are tied individually from distal to proximal. The examination with the patient under anesthesia is repeated with the arthroscope placed first in the posterior central portal, and then in the proximal anterior medial portal, whereas the PLRI pivot shift test is performed to evaluate the adequacy of the reconstruction. Laxity or subluxation still present after the sutures are pretensioned can be corrected by placing an anchor at the isometric point of the lateral epicondyle (as in the acute repairs). One limb of suture is passed under all of the loops of the plication sutures to a retriever and is then brought back over the plicated sutures to pull the entire plicated complex back to the humerus. This is usually noted as part of the preoperative planning and is accomplished before the plication sutures are tied.

POSTOPERATIVE MANAGEMENT

In acute and chronic cases, the patient's elbow is placed in a splint or brace in approximately 30° of extension to relax tension on the repair. Fluoroscopy or radiographs should be used to check the reduction after the splint is applied, as additional flexion may be necessary to tighten the reconstruction and keep the joint reduced. The first postoperative visit usually takes place within 3 to 5 days of the surgery, and the patient's elbow is placed into a hinged brace that allows comfortable movement,

usually 0° to 45°. Shoulder, periscapular, wrist, and hand exercises are initiated and allowed as long as they do not produce pain in the elbow. The patient is seen at 2-week intervals, and motion is slowly increased as much as pain and swelling allow. Once the repair begins to mature, usually between 5 and 8 weeks, physical therapy is increased to include more aggressive upper extremity and core exercises with the elbow brace in place. Normal motion of the elbow is expected by 8 weeks postoperatively, if not earlier. Depending on individual progression, patients are allowed to start strengthening exercises out of the brace at 10 to 12 weeks. They must be able to perform all strengthening exercises pain free in the brace before progression to exercising out of the brace.

OPEN TECHNIQUE

The open technique for plication and repair is similar to that described by O'Driscoll and colleagues. After a diagnostic arthroscopy confirms the instability and the absence of associated pathology, an extensile posterolateral approach is used, and the anconeus muscle is split or retracted anteriorly to access the RUHL complex. The ligaments are plicated and then repaired back to the humerus, as described in the previous section on arthroscopic repair, if adequate tissue is found to allow repair. In revision surgery, or in patients with inadequate tissue for repair, a palmaris autograft or gracilis allograft may be used to reconstruct the joint. The supinator crest of the ulna just posterior to the radial neck is dissected free and the insertion site identified. A 4- to 6- mm tunnel is created in this spot. A Beath pin

Table 1
Comparison of Andrews-Carson Scores

Andrews-Carson Scores	Subjective		Objective		Overall		Average Follow-up (mo)
	Preop	Postop	Preop	Postop	Preop	Postop	
Arthroscopic	55	83	91	93	146	176	33
Open	58	86	86	96	144	182	44
Total	57	85	88	95	145	180	41

is drilled from this point out the ulnar side of the ulna and used to pull a passing suture out this side of the arm. The midportion of the graft is then pulled into the ulna and fixed using an interference screw technique. The two free graft limbs are then brought superiorly, pulling one under the annular ligament and one over the ligament, and attached to the isometric point on the posterior aspect of the lateral epicondyle. The graft should be slightly lax in extension and should tighten with flexion (**Fig. 10**).

PATIENT DATA: MATERIAL AND METHODS

A retrospective chart review was performed for all patients with elbow instability treated surgically by Savoie and Field. About 61 patients with posterolateral elbow reconstructions were identified. Of those patients treated operatively, 54 (89%) had complete data available for review. All patients were evaluated for Andrews-Carson score, length of follow-up, surgical technique used (open vs arthroscopic), age, sex, and previous elbow surgery.[9]

RESULTS

All 54 patients had a PLRI repair, plication, or graft performed. Among them, 41 patients (20

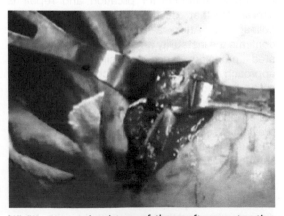

Fig. 10. Anatomic picture of the graft reconstruction for PLRI.

arthroscopic and 21 open) had a combined plication and repair, 10 patients (6 open and 4 arthroscopic) had acute or subacute repairs for recurrent elbow instability, and 3 patients (all open) were reconstructed with a free tendon graft. Ten of the 20 arthroscopically treated patients and 11 of the 21 open plication/repair patients had the addition of an anchor to supplement the arthroscopic suture plication.

The average follow-up was 41 months (range, 12 to 103 months) (**Table 1**). Overall Andrews-Carson scores for all repairs improved from 145 to 180 ($P<.0001$).[9] Subjective scores improved from 57 to 85 ($P<.0001$) and objective scores improved from 88 to 95 ($P = .008$). Subdividing the technique yielded these overall results: arthroscopic repairs improved from 146 to 176 ($P = .0001$), and open repairs from 144 to 182 ($P<.001$). Acute repairs seemed to perform the best, with 9 of 10 patients returning to normal activities, and one to near normal. There was no statistical difference between the results of open versus arthroscopic repair.

SUMMARY

The diagnosis of PLRI is made by a combination of positive clinical findings and radiologic confirmation and may be supplemented by arthroscopic confirmation of instability, including varus opening, the arthroscopic "drive-through sign" of the elbow, and abnormal movement of the radial head and proximal radioulnar joint on the humerus. The posterolateral pivot shift test described by O'Driscoll and colleagues may be performed with the patient supine and prone, and combined with the internal rotation push-up and chair lift tests of Regan and Lapner, gives a clear clinical picture of instability.[1,6] Instability findings may coexist with the standard examination findings of lateral epicondylitis, radial tunnel, and posterolateral plica syndrome. As noted by Kalainov and Cohen, PLRI may actually be a cause of these other elbow problems.[5] About 25% of patients in this study had previous surgery for chronic, recurrent lateral epicondylitis. The authors believe that uncorrected posterolateral instability of the elbow may result in increased tension on the lateral musculature, as it attempts to stabilize the elbow, thereby producing secondary lateral epicondylitis. Other tertiary findings, such as an inflamed posterolateral plica and inflammation of the posterior interosseous nerve in or near the radial tunnel, may also occur with the instability. A high index of suspicion for the instability is necessary to fully evaluate the elbow of patients with all of these findings. The clinical examination recommended by O'Driscoll and by Regan and Lapner certainly will assist in the determination of a coexisting instability as a base cause of these other problems in the elbow.

Additionally, the data suggest that the close proximity of the extensor carpi radialis brevis to the RUHL and lateral collateral ligament complex during lateral epicondylitis procedures may potentially contribute to the iatrogenic development of PLRI. In performing a standard extensor carpi radialis brevis release and repair for recalcitrant lateral epicondylitis, one must remain on the anterior aspect of the lateral epicondyle to avoid damage to the RUHL.

In most patients, repair and plication, whether open or arthroscopic, seemed to be an effective method of managing the instability. Although grafting was necessary in only three of the patients in this study, one should always be prepared to use a supplemental graft. The authors used a semitendinosus allograft in their patients with satisfactory results. It was found that the number of previous surgeries and the time from the initial injury to definitive treatment were the best predictors of the need for a graft. However, low numbers prevent any meaningful recommendation of this technique.

In summary, the authors have described 4 clinical tests for PL instability: (1) supine pivot shift, (2) prone pivot shift, (3) internal rotation wall push-up, and (4) chair push-up. MR arthrography has been recommended to assist in the preoperative evaluation. In surgical cases, arthroscopic confirmation of instability by the "elbow drive-through sign" from the posterior portal and the abnormal movement of the radial head and proximal radial ulnohumeral articulation on the humeral capitellum, while being viewed from the proximal anterior medial portal, confirm the presence of the instability. Finally, the authors described a repair and a ligament plication technique that can be performed either by arthroscopic or by open technique, with a high rate of success.

The study shows that arthroscopic repair and/or plication of the RUHL complex can be as successful as open repair. Arthroscopic repair and suture plication has become a useful technique in shoulder instability, and this report shows that the same ideas can translate to the elbow. The technique is technically demanding and requires a thorough understanding of elbow anatomy. Despite these limitations and concerns, it is thought that arthroscopic repair/plication of the RUHL can effectively stabilize an elbow with PLRI, producing a high degree of patient satisfaction.

REFERENCES

1. O'Driscoll SW, Bell DF, Morrey BF. Posterolateral rotatory instability of the elbow. J Bone Joint Surg Am 1991;73(3):440–6.
2. Dunning CE, Zarzour ZD, Patterson SD, et al. Ligamentous stabilizers against posterolateral rotator instability of the elbow. J Bone Joint Surg Am 2001; 83-A(12):1823–8.
3. Seki A, Olsen BS, Jensen SL, et al. Functional anatomy of the lateral collateral ligament complex of the elbow: configuration of Y and its role. J Shoulder Elbow Surg 2002;11(1):53–9.
4. Smith JP, Savoie FH, Field LD. Posterolateral rotatory instability of the elbow. Clin Sports Med 2001;20(1): 47–58.
5. Kalainov DM, Cohen MS. Posterolateral rotatory instability of the elbow in association with lateral epicondylitis. A report of three cases. J Bone Joint Surg Am 2005;87(5):1120–5.
6. Regan W, Lapner PC. Prospective evaluation of two diagnostic apprehension signs for posterolateral instability of the elbow. J Shoulder Elbow Surg 2006;15(3):344–6.
7. Yadao MA, Savoie FH, Field LD. Posterolateral rotator instability of the elbow. Instr Course Lect 2004;53: 607–14.
8. Potter HG, Weiland AJ, Schatz JA, et al. Posterolateral rotator instability of the elbow: usefulness of MR imaging in diagnosis. Radiology 1997;204(1):185–9.
9. Andrews JR, Carson WG. Arthroscopy of the elbow. Arthroscopy 1985;1(2):97–107.

Open and Arthroscopic Management of Lateral Epicondylitis in the Athlete

Mark S. Cohen, MD[a],*, Anthony A. Romeo, MD[b]

KEYWORDS

• Elbow • Tennis • Epicondylitis • Arthroscopy

"The etiology of tennis elbow is various, its pathology is obscure and its cure is uncertain,"

—*Kellogg Speed, 1929*[1]

Lateral epicondylitis is the most common affliction of the elbow. It was originally described as an occupational condition in the late 1800s.[2,3] The term "tennis elbow" was coined in 1883, because of the association of lateral elbow pain with lawn tennis.[4] Although there has been much effort to identify the etiology and pathology of epicondylitis during the past century, the quote by Speed, delivered in an address to the Royal Society of Medicine, remains relevant today.

From epidemiologic studies, it is clear that epicondylitis most commonly affects individuals of middle age, between 35 and 60 years. It occurs 4 to 5 times as frequently in males as in females and more commonly in the dominant arm.[5,6] It is less common in black individuals.[7] The condition typically begins insidiously, although it is not uncommonly attributed to 1 event or activity. Lateral elbow pain is the most characteristic feature, commonly associated with diminished grip strength. Symptoms are aggravated by activities involving wrist extension against resistance or with applied load.

The pathology of epicondylitis has been attributed to a variety of conditions, including bursitis, synovitis, degenerative arthritis, and so on. The tendinous origin of the extensor carpi radialis brevis (ECRB), however, is the most commonly identified source of pathology.[8,9] Although imaging is not typically required to confirm the diagnosis, abnormal signal of the tendon origin has been confirmed by MR scanning.[10,11] Although irritation of the posterior interosseous nerve can coexist, this is fairly rare.

The source of elbow pain associated with the lateral epicondylitis is poorly understood. Histologic studies have failed to identify inflammation of the extensor tendon origin. However, periostitis of the humeral epicondyle was identified microscopically as early as 1910.[8,12] In addition, reactive granulation tissue containing nerve fibers has been reported in the subtendinous space beneath the ECRB in individuals with this condition.[13] Tendon degeneration (tendinosis) has also been cited as a potential source of pain.[14]

In most cases, lateral epicondylitis is self-limiting, clearing within 8 to 12 months. A variety of conservative measures have been reported to be beneficial, including various therapy modalities, counterforce bracing, acupuncture, and so on.[15] At present, there is insufficient scientific evidence to support any of these treatment methods.[16,17] It is clear that stretching and exercise conditioning are beneficial as opposed to immobilization.[18] Cortisone injection to the epicondyle does provide short-term benefit, although it may not alter the natural history of the condition.[19,20] Once

[a] Section of Hand and Elbow Surgery, Department of Orthopaedic Surgery, Rush University Medical Center, 1725 West Harrison Street, Suite 1063, Chicago, IL 60612, USA
[b] Section of Shoulder Surgery, Department of Orthopaedic Surgery, Rush University Medical Center, 1725 West Harrison Street, Suite 1063, Chicago, IL 60612, USA
* Corresponding author.
E-mail address: mcohen3@rush.edu (M.S. Cohen).

Hand Clin 25 (2009) 331–338
doi:10.1016/j.hcl.2009.05.003
0749-0712/09/$ – see front matter © 2009 Published by Elsevier Inc.

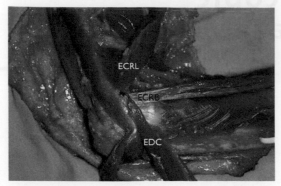

Fig. 1. Anatomic specimen (*right elbow*) with the extensor tendon origins dissected. The ECRL is reflected anteriorly, and the extensor digitorum communis posteriorly, to reveal the ECRB tendon.

epicondylitis resolves, recurrence is rare, and it has been reported in less than 3% of cases.[21]

ANATOMY

The extensor carpi radialis longus (ECRL) and the ECRB have a unique relationship at the level of the elbow (**Fig. 1**). The ECRL origin is entirely muscular along the lateral supracondylar ridge of the humerus. The muscle origin has a triangular configuration, with the apex pointing proximally. In contrast, the origin of the ECRB is entirely tendinous. Although it blends with the origin of the

extensor digitorum communis (EDC), when dissected from a distal to proximal direction, using the tendon undersurface, it can be separated from the EDC back to the humerus.[22] The anatomic origin of the ECRB is located just beneath the distal-most tip of the lateral supracondylar ridge. The footprint is diamond shaped, measuring approximately 13 × 7 mm (**Fig. 2**). At the level of the radiocapitellar joint, the ECRB is intimate with the underlying anterior capsule of the elbow joint, but it is easily separable at this level.[22]

OPERATIVE TREATMENT: OPEN METHODS

Surgery is reportedly required in approximately 4% to 8% of cases.[7,21,23] However, this probably represents a falsely high estimate, as the denominator is likely greater because of those individuals who do not seek formal medical evaluation. The first effective surgical procedure reported for lateral epicondylitis dates back to 1873. Runge[3] used simple cautery to burn all tissue from the skin down to the humerus. Since that time, several surgical procedures have been described, including simple resection of the epicondyle, resection of the annular ligament and joint synovium, percutaneous or open division of the common extensor origin, distal tendon lengthening, denervation, radial nerve decompression, and epicondylar resection followed by aconeous

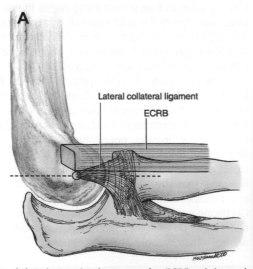

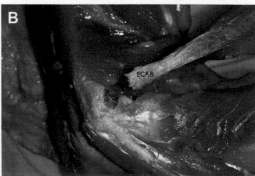

Fig. 2. (*A*) Relationship between the ECRB origin at the humerus and bony landmarks. Note that the ECRB footprint origin is diamond shaped and located between the midline of the joint and the top of the humeral capitellum beneath the most distal extent of the supracondylar ridge. The tendon does not originate on the epicondyle specifically. Note the relationship between the ECRB origin and the underlying lateral collateral ligament. (*B*) Lateral view of cadaveric specimen. The ECRL and EDC have been removed, revealing the ECRB footprint on the humerus. (*From* Cohen MS, Romeo AA, Hennigan SP, et al. Lateral epicondylitis: anatomic relationships of the extensor tendon origins and implications for arthroscopic treatment. J Shoulder Elbow Surg 2008;17(6):959; with permission.)

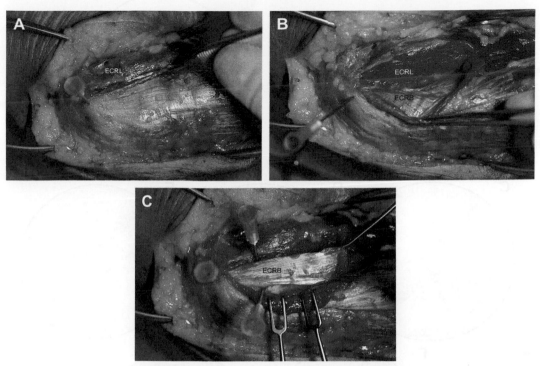

Fig. 3. (*A*) Cadaveric specimen depicting the junction between the muscular ECRL anteriorly and the extensor aponeurosis posteriorly, which has been opened. (*B*) The aponeurosis and tendons have been reflected posteriorly off of the ECRL, revealing the undersurface of the ECRB tendon. (*C*) The EDC has been dissected off of the underlying ECRB, revealing the anterior and posterior margins of the ECRB tendon.

coverage.[16,24–26] All methods have been reported to provide successful outcomes.

The most common technique used involves identification and excision of any abnormally identified tissue at the extensor tendon origin with creation of a bony bed to promote healing, followed by reapproximation of the overlying aponeurosis. The procedure requires identification of the ECRB tendon. The bony origin of the extensor brevis is beneath the lateral epicondylar prominence, along a longitudinally oriented ridge, coursing from the top of the capitellum to the midline of the radiocapitellar joint (see **Fig. 1**).

Distal to the epicondyle, the ECRB tendon lies beneath the EDC and its aponeurosis. It can most easily be identified by dissecting in an anterior to posterior direction, beginning at the junction between the ECRL and EDC aponeurosis (**Fig. 3**). The undersurface of the brevis tendon can be elevated from the longus muscle in oblique fashion. The aponeurosis of the EDC lies on top of the brevis and is tightly opposed.

An alternative method of brevis tendon identification involves anterior elevation of the common tendon origin beginning at the midline of the radiocapitellar joint (**Fig. 4**). This marks the posterior margin of the brevis tendon. Elevation posterior to the midline of the joint is unnecessary and puts the collateral ligament complex origin in jeopardy. The brevis undersurface is debrided, and the epicondylar origin is denuded or drilled. The fascia is then closed.

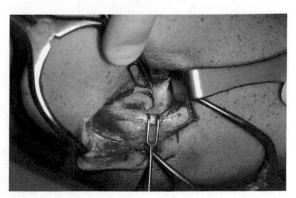

Fig. 4. Intraoperative photograph of a right elbow depicting elevation of ECRB origin from the humeral epicondyle. Dissection is begun at the midline of the radiocapitellar joint. Drill holes have been made in the humerus to promote healing.

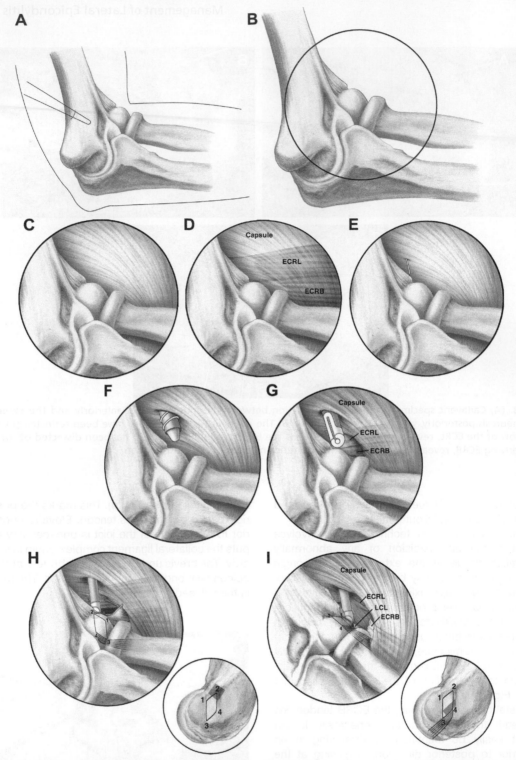

Fig. 5. (*A*) Medial portal used in visualization for the arthroscopic lateral epicondylar release. (*B* and *C*) Field of view from the medial portal. (*D*) Relationship of the extensor tendon origins when viewed intraarticularly. They are located outside (behind) the elbow capsule. (*E*) Needle used to help establish a modified lateral portal. Note how this is begun slightly proximal and anterior to the proximal margin of the humeral capitellum. (*F*) Cannula used to establish the final lateral portal. (*G*) Release of the capsule from the lateral humeral margin allowing visualization of the tendinous origins behind. The ECRL is more anteriorly located and is muscular. The ECRB is more posterior. (*H*) The ECRB is released from the top of the capitellum to the (*I*) midline of the radiocapitellar joint. (*Courtesy* of Mark S. Cohen, MD, Chiacogo, IL; with permission.)

OPERATIVE TREATMENT: ARTHROSCOPIC METHODS

There has been interest in the surgical treatment of lateral epicondylitis from within the joint using arthroscopic methods. Cited advantages include the ability to debride the brevis tendon undersurface without division of the common extensor aponeurosis, the ability to evaluate the joint for intraarticular pathology, and possibly a shortened rehabilitation.[27,28]

The procedure requires a familiarity with arthroscopic instrumentation and techniques as applied to the elbow joint. The authors favor the prone position. Bony landmarks are drawn out, and a standard anteromedial portal is established (**Fig. 5**). This is started several centimeters proximal and anterior to the medial epicondyle and well anterior to the palpable intermuscular septum. Care is taken to slide along the anterior humerus, and the joint is entered with a blunt introducer or a switching stick. This medial portal allows one to view the lateral joint, including the radial head, capitellum, and the lateral capsule. It is often helpful at this point to open the inflow to allow distension of the capsule. If visualization is a problem, a retractor can be introduced through a proximal anterolateral portal 2 to 3 cm proximal and just anterior to the lateral supracondylar ridge. A simple Freer elevator is useful for this purpose. By tensioning the capsule anteriorly, improved visualization of the lateral capsule and soft tissues can be achieved.

A modified anterolateral portal is established using an inside-out technique. This is started 2 to 3 cm above and anterior to the lateral epicondyle (see **Fig. 5**). The portal is slightly more proximal than a standard anterolateral portal. This allows instrumentation down to the tendon origin rather than entering the joint through the ECRB tendon itself. If lateral synovitis is present, this can be debrided with a resector.

The capsule is next released. Occasionally in epicondylitis, one can find a disruption of the underlying capsule from the humerus (**Fig. 6**). Most commonly, the capsule is intact, although small linear tears can be present (**Fig. 7**). The authors have found it easier to release the lateral soft tissues in layers using a monopolar thermal device. In this way, the capsule is first incised or released from the humerus. When it retracts distally, one can appreciate the ECRB tendon posteriorly and the ECRL, which is principally muscular, more anteriorly.

Once the capsule is adequately resected, the ECRB origin is released from the epicondyle (see **Figs. 5** and **7**). This is started at the top of the

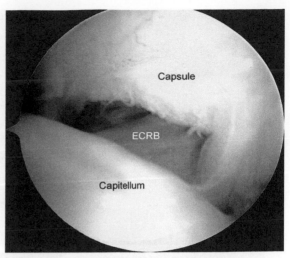

Fig. 6. Initial intraoperative view of a patient with recalcitrant lateral epicondylitis. Note the capsular rent. In some cases, the capsule is noted to have torn away from its humeral origin.

capitellum and carried posteriorly. The lateral collateral ligament is not at risk if the release is kept anterior to the midline of the radiocapitellar joint.[29] On average, adequate resection of the ECRB must include approximately 13 mm of tendon origin from anterior to posterior.[22] Care is taken to drive in the scope adequately to view the release down to the midline of the radiocapitellar joint. Typically, the entire ECRB retracts distally away from the humerus.

After the ECRB is detached, one should be careful not to release the extensor aponeurosis, which lies behind the ECRB tendon. This can be visualized as a stripped background of transversely (longitudinally) oriented tendon and muscular fibers, much less distinct than the ECRB (see **Fig. 7**). It is located posterior to the ECRL, which again is principally muscular in origin. If the aponeurosis is violated, one will debride into the subcutaneous tissue about the lateral elbow.

DISCUSSION

The majority of retrospective studies report successful outcomes after surgical intervention, with good (80%–90%) and excellent results.[23,30] The largest prospective series, however, consisting of 57 patients followed for approximately 5 years after an open procedure, revealed continued symptoms in many patients.[31] In this study, moderate to severe pain was reported in 40% of patients at 6 weeks postoperatively and in 24% at 1 year. At 5 years, although most surgically treated patients were improved, 9% continued to

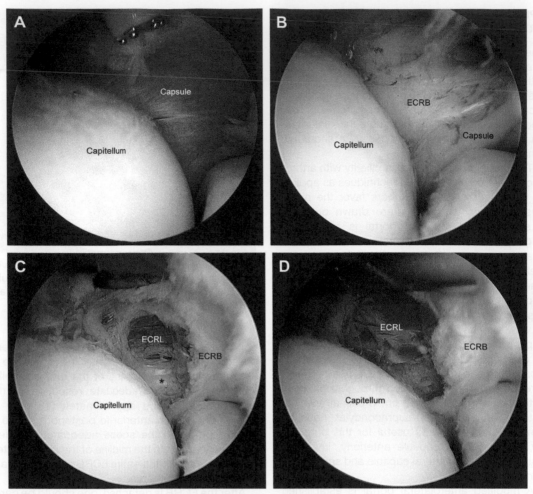

Fig. 7. (*A*) Initial intraoperative view of a patient treated surgically for lateral epicondylitis. The lateral capsule obstructs the view of the extensor tendon origins. Note the small longitudinal rent in the capsule. (*B*) The capsule has been released, revealing the muscular ECRL anteriorly and the tendinous ECRB more posteriorly. Note the capsular layer distally, which is deep to the tendon. (*C*) The ECRB has been released. Behind this, one can see the muscular ECRL anteriorly and the extensor aponeurosis that lies behind the ECRB (*asterisk*). It is characteristically composed of longitudinally stripped tendinous fibers much less distinct than the ECRB. (*D*) Final close-up view after ECRB release. Using the resector, one can see the thick ECRB origin that has retracted distally following release.

experience moderate to severe pain, and 28% reported persistent low-grade symptoms.

Of late, there has been an interest in arthroscopic treatment of lateral epicondylitis.[29,32–36] A cadaveric study demonstrated that arthroscopic release of the ECRB was a safe, reliable, and reproducible procedure for refractory lateral epicondylitis.[28] However, the results of arthroscopic treatment of this condition have been variable. Tseng[36] reported satisfactory results in 9 of 11 patients. However, he also had a 33% complication rate. Stapleton and Baker[35] compared 5 patients treated arthroscopically with 10 patients treated by open debridement. They reported similar results and complication rates between the two groups. Later, Baker and colleagues[32] reported on 39 elbows treated arthroscopically, with 37 reporting being "better" or "much better" at follow-up. Peart and colleagues[34] reported on 33 arthroscopic procedures for lateral epicondylitis with 28% of patients failing to achieve good or excellent outcomes.

The authors reviewed a consecutive series of 36 patients with recalcitrant lateral epicondylitis treated with arthroscopic release using the aforementioned technique.[37] There were 24 men and 12 women with an average age of 42 years at the time of surgery. The cohort had symptoms for an average of 19 months before surgical intervention. Intraoperative findings revealed significant lateral intraarticular synovitis in approximately 30% of patients. All patients were evaluated by independent examiners at a minimum 2-year follow-up. On average, patients required 4 weeks to return to regular activities and 7 weeks to return to sports and full work duties. No major complications were reported. One patient had a neurapraxia of the superficial radial nerve that resolved by 2 weeks postoperatively. The average functional component of the Mayo Elbow Performance Score at follow-up averaged 11.1 out of 12 (range, 5 to 12). Grip strength averaged 91% of the opposite, uninvolved side. Subjective pain ratings as measured on a visual analog scale improved from 8.5 ± 2.4 to 1.9 ± 1.3 (P<.01). However, 10 patients reported continued pain with strenuous activities and repetitive use of the affected arm. Two patients continued to have significant pain and were considered failures.[37]

From a review of the literature, it is clear that surgical intervention for lateral epicondylitis is somewhat less predictable than other operative procedures about the elbow. No variables predictive of success have been identified, including time between the onset of symptoms and surgery, occupation, grip strength, severity of pain, limitation of motion, tenderness, age, number of cortisone injections, and the use of preoperative therapy.[31] When surgery is offered, patients must be counseled on the possibility of a long recovery period, with some continued symptoms about the lateral elbow. Arthroscopic release may offer a more rapid return of function. Knowledge of the anatomy, including the extensor tendon origins, is essential for effective surgical release regardless of the technique used.

REFERENCES

1. Speed K. Tennis elbow. BMJ 1929;2(1):122–3.
2. Bernhardt M. Ueber eine wenig bekannte Form der Beschaftigungsneuralgie. Neurol Centralblatt 1896; 15:13–6 [In German].
3. Runge F. Zur Genese und Behandlung des Schreibekrampfes. Berliner Klin Wchnschr 1873;10:245–8 [In German].
4. Major HP. Lawn-tennis elbow. Br Med J 1883;2: 557–64.
5. Garden RS. Tennis elbow. J Bone Joint Surg Br 1961;43B:100–6.
6. Gruchow HW, Pelletier D. An epidemiologic study of tennis elbow. Incidence, recurrence and effectiveness of preventive strategies. Am J Sports Med 1979;7:234–8.
7. Coonrad RW, Hooper R. Tennis elbow: its course, natural history, conservative and surgical management. J Bone Joint Surg 1973;55A:1177–82.
8. Cyriax JH. The pathology and treatment of tennis elbow. J Bone Joint Surg 1936;18:921–40.
9. Regan W, Wold LE, Coonrad R, et al. Microscopic histopathology of chronic refractory lateral epicondylitis. Am J Sports Med 1992;20:746–9.
10. Ho CP. MR imaging of tendon injuries in the elbow. Magn Reson Imaging Clin N Am 1997;5:529–43.
11. Martin CE, Schweitzer ME. MR imaging of epicondylitis. Skeletal Radiol 1998;27:133–8.
12. Franke F. Ueber epicondylitis humeri. Dtsch Med Wochenschr 1910;36:13–9 [In German].
13. Goldie I. Epicondylitis lateralis humeri (epicondylalgia or tennis elbow): a pathological study. Acta Chir Scand Suppl 1964;339:1–119.
14. Kraushaar BS, Nirschl RP. Tendinosis of the elbow: clinical features and findings of histological, immunohistochemical and electron microscopy studies. J Bone Joint Surg 1999;81A:259–78.
15. Galloway M, DeMaio M, Mangine R. Rehabilitation techniques in the treatment of medial and lateral epicondylitis. Orthopedics 1992;15:1089–96.
16. Boyer MI, Hastings H. Lateral tennis elbow: "Is there any science out there?". J Shoulder Elbow Surg 1999;8:481–91.
17. Labelle H, Guibert R, Joncas J, et al. Lack of scientific evidence for the treatment of lateral epicondylitis of the elbow. An attempted meta-analysis. J Bone Joint Surg Br 1992;74:646–51.
18. Pienimaki T, Karinen P, Kemila T, et al. Long-term follow-up of conservatively treated chronic tennis elbow patients. A prospective and retrospective analysis. Scand J Rehabil Med 1998;30:159–66.
19. Assendelft WJ, Hay EM, Adshead R, et al. Corticosteroid injections for lateral epicondyltis: a systematic overview. Br J Gen Pract 1996;46:209–16.
20. Hay EM, Paterson SM, Lewis M, et al. Pragmatic randomized controlled trial of local corticosteroid injection and naproxen for treatment of lateral epicondylitis of elbow in primary care. BMJ 1999;319: 964–8.
21. Boyd HB, McLeod AC. Tennis elbow. J Bone Joint Surg 1973;55A:1183–7.
22. Cohen MS, Romeo AA, Hennigan SP, et al. Lateral epicondylitis: anatomic relationships of the extensor tendon origins and implications for arthroscopic treatment. J Shoulder Elbow Surg 2008;17(6): 954–60.
23. Nirschl RP, Pettrone FA. The surgical treatment of lateral epicondylitis. J Bone Joint Surg 1979;61A: 832–9.
24. Almquist EE, Necking L, Bach AW. Epicondylar resection with anconeus muscle transfer for chronic lateral epicondyltis. J Hand Surg Am 1998;23: 723–31.
25. Bosworth DM. Surgical treatment of tennis elbow: a follow-up study. J Bone Joint Surg 1965;47A: 1533–6.

26. Posch JH, Goldberg VM, Larrey R. Extensor fasciotomy for tennis elbow: a long-term follow-up study. Clin Orthop 1978;135:179–82.

27. Baker CL. Arthroscopic versus open techniques for extensor tendinosis of the elbow. Tech Shoulder Elbow Surg 2000;1:184–91.

28. Kuklo TR, Taylor KF, Murphy KP, et al. Arthroscopic release for lateral epicondylitis: a cadaveric model. Arthroscopy 1999;15:259–64.

29. Smith AM, Castle JA, Ruch DS. Arthroscopic resection of the common extensor origin: anatomic considerations. J Shoulder Elbow Surg 2003;12(4):375–9.

30. Morrey BF. Surgical failure of tennis elbow. In: Morrey BF, editor. The elbow and its disorders. 3rd edition. Philadelphia: W.B. Saunders; 2000. p. 543–8.

31. Verhaar J, Walenkamp G, Kester A, et al. Lateral extensor release for tennis elbow: a prospective long-term study. J Bone Joint Surg 1993;75A: 1034–43.

32. Baker CL, Murphy KP, Gottlob CA, et al. Arthroscopic classification and treatment of lateral epicondylitis: two-year clinical results. J Shoulder Elbow Surg 2000;9(6):475–82.

33. Cummins CA. Lateral epicondylitis: in vivo assessment of arthroscopic debridment and correlation with patient outcomes. Am J Sports Med 2006;34: 1486–91.

34. Peart RE, Strickler SS, Schweitzer. Lateral epicondylitis: a comparative study of open and arthroscopic lateral release. Am J Orthop 2004;33: 565–7.

35. Stapleton TR, Baker CL. Arthroscopic treatment of lateral epicondylitis. Arthroscopy 1996;10:335–6.

36. Tseng V. Arthroscopic lateral release for treatment of tennis elbow. Arthroscopy 1994;10:335–6.

37. Lattermann C, Anbari A, McCarty LP, et al. Three-year follow-up of arthroscopic treatment for recalcitrant lateral epicondylitis. J Shoulder and Elbow Surg [submitted].

Medial Collateral Ligament Reconstruction in the Baseball Pitcher's Elbow

Holger C. Erne, MD[a], Ioannis C. Zouzias, MD[b],
Melvin P. Rosenwasser, MD[c],*

KEYWORDS

- Medial ulnar collateral ligament
- Ulnar collateral ligament • Thrower's elbow
- Baseball injuries • "Tommy John" surgery

Elbow problems in overhead-throwing athletes were first reported in 1941 among professional baseball players.[1] Five years later, Waris[2] described the injury to the medial ulnar collateral ligament (MCL) from valgus forces in 17 elite javelin throwers. Since that time, the MCL has been studied by many sports medicine specialists. By virtue of the numbers of participants, baseball, especially pitching, has been most frequently associated with injury to this important ligament. The procedure described by Jobe and colleagues,[3] with reconstruction of the MCL, has been modified to decrease soft tissue morbidity to the flexor pronator origin and the ulnar nerve.

ANATOMY

The MCL complex of the elbow is composed of three discrete portions: the anterior bundle, the posterior bundle, and the oblique bundle (transverse ligament). The anterior bundle inserts onto the sublime tubercle of the medial coronoid process and is the most prime stabilizer against valgus stress of the elbow joint.[4] The anterior bundle courses an average of 4.7 mm from the anterior-inferior medial epicondyle of the humerus and inserts distally on the ulnohumeral articulation of the sublime tubercle. It has an average

thickness of 2.7 mm. The anterior ligament itself has two parts that function in a reciprocal fashion.[4] The anterior band of the anterior bundle is taut from 30° to 90° of flexion, whereas the posterior band is taut from 60° to 120° of flexion. The anterior band is more vulnerable to valgus stress with the elbow extended, whereas the posterior band is more vulnerable with the elbow flexed. The posterior bundle of the MCL is thinner and weaker compared with the anterior bundle. It is fan shaped and originates from the inferior portion of the medial epicondyle and inserts on the medial margin of the semilunar notch. The posterior bundle provides secondary restraint at flexion beyond 90°.[4–6] It has been shown to be vulnerable to valgus stress only when the anterior bundle is insufficient.[7] The oblique bundle serves to expand the greater sigmoid notch as a thickening of the joint capsule extending from the medial olecranon to the inferior medial coronoid process.[8] It does not cross the elbow joint.

PATHOPHYSIOLOGY

Pitching is stressful and increases the valgus moment and force on the MCL. The pitching motion has been divided into four stages: windup, cocking, acceleration, and follow-through. The transition

[a] Handchirurgie Rhoen-Klink, Salzburger Leite 1, 97616 Bad Neustadt/Saale, Germany
[b] Department of Orthopedic Surgery, New York Presbyterian Hospital, Columbia University Medical Center, 622 West 168th Street, New York, NY 10032, USA
[c] New York Presbyterian Hospital, Columbia University Medical Center, 622 West 168th Street, Room 1150, New York, NY 10032, USA
* Corresponding author.
E-mail address: mpr2@columbia.edu (M.P. Rosenwasser).

Hand Clin 25 (2009) 339–346
doi:10.1016/j.hcl.2009.05.006
0749-0712/09/$ – see front matter © 2009 Published by Elsevier Inc.

from cocking phase to acceleration phase occurs when the shoulder is at a point of maximal external rotation. At the late cocking phase, maximal force is applied to the medial elbow and resisted by the MCL.[9,10] The moment of inertia experienced at the medial elbow during maximal external rotation of the shoulder is calculated at 64 N m.[11] According to Morrey,[12] when the elbow is in 90° of flexion, the MCL assumes 54% of this valgus moment, about 34 N m. Two studies have shown that the ultimate load to failure of the native MCL is estimated at 34 N m.[10,11] Therefore, the forces experienced by the native MCL during overhead-throwing approach the tensile limit. Continued pitching can lead to overload and soft tissue microtrauma with ligament attenuation and ultimately ligament rupture. As the medial ligament degenerates, the kinematics of the elbow are changed with increased valgus rotation of the ulnohumeral joint. This repetitive deceleration and focal impact cause the posterior medial olecranon to impinge on the medial crista of the distal humerus and is called the "valgus extension overload syndrome." This clinical picture is seen in 16% to 45% of patients requiring MCL reconstruction.[13]

HISTORY

Injury to the MCL can be acute or chronic. In an acute rupture, the athlete may describe a sudden onset of medial elbow pain while throwing, sometimes with an audible pop, and cannot resume pitching. Chronic ligament injuries appear as persistent low-level medial elbow pain during the late cocking and early acceleration phase of throwing. Although the athlete can still throw, he has decreased command and velocity, as reported in 50% of athletes by Conway and colleagues.[14] MCL instability may cause cubital tunnel syndrome or local syndromes with distal radiation. Mechanical ulnar nerve symptoms can be attributed to reactive synovitis of the medial joint adjacent to the nerve and may be associated with hypertrophy of the medial intermuscular septum. Pitchers may experience pain at terminal extension or follow-through because of osteophytes and cartilage damage, with or without the presence of loose chondral bodies. This is known as posterior humeroulna impingement.

PHYSICAL EXAMINATION

The examination for MCL injury is reproducible in the setting of complete rupture with focal pain and instability but inconsistent in attenuation injuries. Focal tenderness of the MCL at its insertion into the coronoid and pain on hyperextension

are often noted. Mobility is usually full for flexion but may be limited 2° to 5° of terminal extension secondary to osteophytes (**Fig. 1**). Ulnar nerve tenderness can be found not only at the cubital tunnel but also proximally along the medial intermuscular septum. Some pitchers may present clinical signs of radial tunnel entrapment syndrome at the arcade of Frohse manifested by local pain only. The presence of joint effusion is common if osteochondral loose bodies are present. MCL instability can be assessed by various clinical tests. They include the valgus stress test, the "milking maneuver," and the moving valgus stress test. The valgus stress test is performed with the shoulder held in abduction and external rotation. The examiner stabilizes the arm and flexes the elbow to 30° to unlock the ulnohumeral joint. A valgus stress is then placed on the elbow (**Fig. 2**). The test is positive if the patient has pain or apprehension of instability. The "milking maneuver" is performed by extending and externally rotating the humerus to neutralize glenohumeral motion. The forearm is then supinated and a valgus stress is applicated to the elbow by extending the thumb with the elbow flexed at 90°. The examiner palpates along the course of the MCL. This test stresses the ligament and isolates the anterior bundle of the MCL but is not entirely reliable, given the high rate of false positives. Lastly, the moving valgus stress test is essentially a dynamic milking maneuver. It was first described by O'Driscoll and colleagues.[15] This test has been shown to be highly sensitive (100%) and specific (75%) for elbow pain that is directly related to injury of the MCL. The patient's arm is placed in the same position as the milking maneuver, but a constant valgus stress is placed at the elbow as it is moved rapidly through the arc of flexion and extension. The test is considered positive if it reproduces the patient's symptoms between 70°

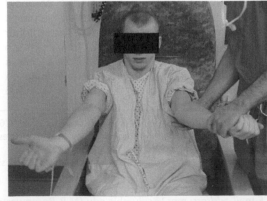

Fig. 1. Range of motion. Patient unable to fully extend elbow (posterior impingement).

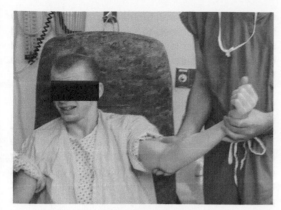

Fig. 2. Positive and painful valgus stress test.

and 120° (shear zone), when the pitcher would feel pain while throwing. All partial injuries are harder to diagnose clinically. Ulnar neuropathy may be associated with MCL pathology, but distal signs must be carefully assessed to rule out concomitant or confounding embolic disease, ulnar neuroma, or subluxation, with documentation of motor and sensory function of the hand.

IMAGING
Plain Radiographs

Radiographs with three views, anterior-posterior, lateral, and oblique are obtained. The lateral view is taken with the elbow at 90°. Many changes, such as loose bodies, osteophytes, and heterotopic calcifications, are assessed, along with occurrence of osteochondritis dissecans. Many pitchers have these findings. Occasionally there is a fracture of a prominent posterior osteophyte or the rare presence of a proximal ulnar (olecranon) stress fracture.

Ultrasonography

To diagnose soft tissue pathology, ultrasound is a fast, noninvasive and cost-effective method in

the hands of an experienced user. The method can provide information about the integrity of the medial collateral ligament in athletes.[16] This technique is not frequently used, as it requires technical expertise.

MRI

MRI best assesses the integrity of the MCL. Modern scanners with dedicated extremity coils provide high-resolution images of the ligament. The anterior bundle of the MCL is best visualized on coronal T1-weighted images, as it is taut in extension.[17] In a cadaver study evaluating the usefulness of thin-section three-dimensional Fourier transform gradient echo imaging, the ligament was best seen on images reformatted into a slightly posterior obliqued coronal plane.[18] In the presence of injury to the MCL, nonhomogeneous, increased signal intensity within and surrounding the anterior bundle of the MCL is noted. These abnormalities are more prominent on T2 weighted images. Loose bodies and osteochondral lesions are best seen on sagittal projections. Image enhancement by way of saline or gadolinium arthrogram is possible but increasingly unnecessary with the use of larger magnets. MR arthrography has been shown to have a sensitivity of 92% for identifying tears of the MCL (**Fig. 3** A, B).[19] In the presence of inner surface partial tears and small full-thickness perforations, fat-suppressed T1-weighted MR arthrography with gadolinium may provide useful information.[18]

Arthroscopy

Elbow arthroscopy is an adjunct to the clinical diagnosis and may confirm the dynamic stress test. It is helpful to inspect the cartilage surfaces and remove osteochondral bodies and osteophytes either anteriorly or posteriorly. If posterior

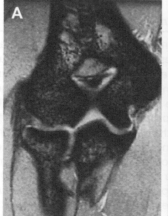
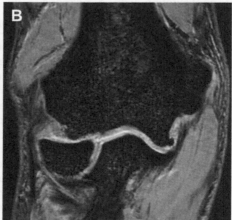

Fig. 3. (A) T-sign on MRI of intrasubstance MCL tear (usual location of injury in pitchers). (B) MCL tear.

impingement is the major source of pain, limited debridement may permit successful return to pitching, although minimal resection is suggested to protect the evolving MCL injury.

TREATMENT
Nonoperative Treatment

Duration of symptoms, age of pitcher, and level of competition are all determinants in the initial course of treatment. All pitchers should have complete rest for 2 to 3 months at first presentation. Rehabilitation includes rotator cuff stretching and strengthening and information on pitching technique. Rettig and colleagues[20] described a nonsurgical protocol with 42% of competitive pitchers returning to competition at the previous level. Scholastic athletes are often encouraged to change positions or sports, but elite high school pitchers and above are evaluated and considered for reconstruction if examination and imaging confirm MCL injury. Time is critical for these athletes, and surgical reconstruction allows resumption of their careers and minimizes loss of season and eligibility when in school.

Operative Treatment

The first published and often cited MCL reconstruction was the one performed by Jobe on pitcher Tommy John, reported in 1986.[3] This case documented the first successful reconstruction of the MCL, which allowed him to continue pitching in the major leagues. His recovery and rehabilitation took 2 years as it was complicated by an ulnar neuropraxia. Jobe and colleagues' initial report describes a common flexor pronator origin release to expose the MCL. The ulnar nerve is then released from the cubital tunnel and transposed anteriorly. Transosseus holes are created in the ulna and medial epicondyle for passage in a figure-of-eight configuration with a palmaris graft. The bone tunnels are sited on the sublime tubercle and medial epicondyle at the anatomic origin and insertion of the MCL. Jobe's technique was modified by Smith and colleagues[21] in 1996, with a muscle-splitting approach through the posterior third of the common flexor bundle. This modification, which maintains the tendinous origin intact, is now universal and still permits ulnar nerve production, tunnel creation, and graft tensioning. In 2002, Rohrbough and Altchek described the docking technique, which advocated an interference screw technique for fixation of the graft within the humeral epicondyle.[22,23] This was advanced to aid in the tensioning and fixation of the graft on the humeral side, and it is especially useful if the palmaris graft is not long enough to emerge from

the superior humeral tunnels to be adequately tensioned.[22] Rohrbough and colleagues used a single palmaris longus graft; others have used double or three-strain technique to increase the tensile strength of the reconstruction.[24,25]

SURGICAL TECHNIQUES
Direct Repair

The authors believe that in throwing athletes there is no role for direct repair of the torn MCL. Repair of a ruptured or attenuated MCL does not support the stresses of pitching, and pitchers can ill afford a failed repair followed by a reconstruction, as more than two seasons would be lost. The poor outcome is well documented in the literature.[14,26]

Muscle Splitting; Flexor-pronator Origin

As noted in the initial report, Jobe and colleagues[3] described a detachment of the flexor-pronator mass. Subsequent reports demonstrate improved outcomes with the muscle-splitting approach.[23] An intact tendinous origin of the important forearm flexors allows early rehabilitation without fear or muscle detachment and allows predictable restoration of full mobility.

Ulnar Nerve Handling

MCL reconstruction combined with routine ulnar nerve transposition yields 15% less excellent results and twice the rate of postoperative neuropathy.[23] The authors recommend an in situ decompression of the ulnar nerve in the cubital tunnel to protect the nerve during tunnel creation and graft passage; they recommend transposition only if the patient had preexisting ulnar nerve symptoms. The authors believe that submuscular transposition is contraindicated in the throwing athlete having MCL reconstruction because of the requisite flexor pronator detachment and subsequent scarring.

Bony Tunnels

Remnants of the MCL at its origin and insertion are preserved to allow precise bone tunnel sitting and to enhance the palmaris longus graft reconstruction with imbricating sutures. The ulnar tunnels are started with a 2.0-mm drill bit and then expanded with larger drills in a stepwise fashion with a 2.5- and 3.5-mm drill bit. This creates concentric holes and lessens potential for stress fractures. Hole spacing must be at least 8 mm at the ulnar tunnels for adequate bony support and to prevent fracture of the bridge during tensioning. The holes for the proximal insertion are prepared using a 2.5-mm drill bit at the inferior medial epicondyle and then diverted along the cortical

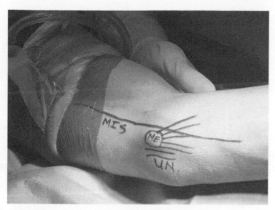

Fig. 4. Incision.

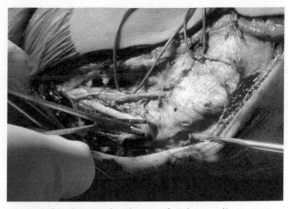

Fig. 6. Cubital tunnel: release of Osborne ligament.

column margin and into a Y configuration, one anterior and one posterior, being careful not to notch or violate the medial column cortex to avoid medial epicondyle fracture. The holes are expanded stepwise with the 3.0- and 3.5-mm drill bit for accuracy and control. The graft should be passed without restriction or fretting, and the dimensions will allow the palmaris longus or extensor digiti communis to be passed and tensioned without difficulty. Care is taken to protect the ulnar nerve during passage.

Graft

The most common graft in the literature is the palmaris longus tendon.[23] Other options are the extensor digiti communis tendon of the toes or one-half of the flexor carpi radialis tendon. The authors' preferred graft is the contralateral palmaris longus tendon to avoid any potential injury to the hand and wrist that grips the baseball. The second choice when palmaris longus is absent is the extensor tendon of the third or fourth toe. The authors do not use split tendons because of the tendency for them to fray or unravel. The graft

must be equally tensioned through all tunnels with a prolonged stretch for preconditioning to minimize any subsequent viscoelastic lengthening.

Authors' Preferred Method

The incision is made straight medial, centered over the epicondyle and extended along the medial epicondylar ridge 4 to 5 cm and distally along the posterior margin of the flexor pronator origin to 2 to 3 cm before the coronoid (**Fig. 4**). The medial antebrachial cutaneous nerve is identified and protected (**Fig. 5**). The ulnar nerve is identified proximal to the cubital tunnel (**Fig. 6**). The cubital tunnel is opened in an antegrade fashion, preserving all motor branches to the flexor carpi ulnaris. A muscle-splitting incision is performed at the flexor pronator origin in midsubstance. The origin is preserved. The deeper tendon investments are dissected from the capsule and the MCL. The sublime tubercle is an easily palpable landmark, and the full width of the footprint of the MCL is identified to help the ulnar tunnel creation (**Fig. 7**). The holes are parallel and orientated superior and inferior by drilling convergently. Graft

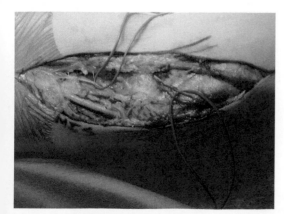

Fig. 5. Superficial dissection.

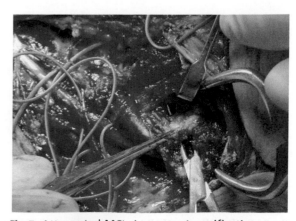

Fig. 7. Attenuated MCL, heterotopic ossification.

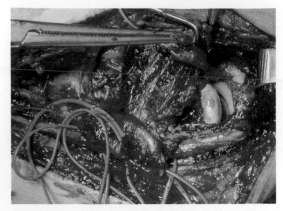

Fig. 8. Elevation of attenuated MCL demonstrates insertion site in sublime tubercle of ulna.

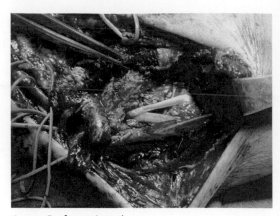

Fig. 10. Graft tensioned.

passage is performed with suture passers attached to the graft. The palmaris longus tendon graft is harvested from the contralateral wrist with a tendon stripper. Great care is taken to identify the palmar cutaneous branch of the median nerve. The median nerve itself should not be visible, but it has been misidentified in the past and harvested, so great care should be taken to prevent this from happening. Any structure with a visible axial blood vessel should not be taken. The tensioning is performed in 90° flexion and neutral angulation to prevent inadvertent valgus at final graft placement (**Fig. 8**). The graft is pulled and tensioned as tight as possible (**Figs. 9** and **10**). The graft is placed in ulnar tunnels first; it is then placed in a figure-of-eight and passed through the epicondyle and tied on the back to itself with multiple points of fixation. The remnant of the previous medial collateral ligament reinforces the graft by imbricating over the tendon graft (**Figs. 11** and **12**).

POSTOPERATIVE REHABILITATION

In Phase I, patients get a hinged elbow orthosis locked at 90° for 2 weeks. After 2 weeks, the orthosis is unlocked, and motion from 30° to unlimited flexion is allowed for 2 weeks. At 4 weeks, unlimited motion is allowed. The orthosis is worn continuously until 6 weeks. At 6 weeks, Phase II, motion usually is full, and forearm strengthening begins. At 12 weeks, Phase III, the athlete is allowed to begin soft long toss exercises, 60 to 90 ft every other day. At 16 weeks, Phase IV, the interval-throwing protocol begins. The athlete is allowed to begin pitching from a 60 ft distance at 50% velocity for 15 to 20 minutes from flat ground every other day. At 24 weeks, conditioning progresses to a pitch count of 30 to 60 pitches or a simulation of two innings, and the pitcher can now throw from a raised mount. From 24 to 36 weeks, the pitch counts and pitch selection are increased, followed by a return to competition if there is no pain or synovitis.

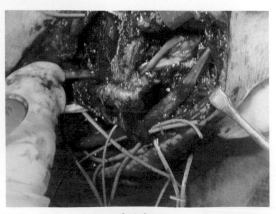

Fig. 9. Graft in figure-of-eight position, tensioning.

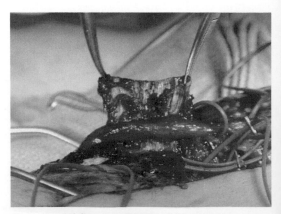

Fig. 11. Fascial flap to prevent subluxation.

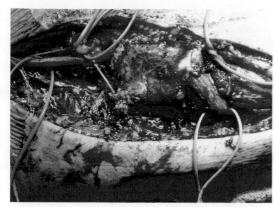

Fig. 12. Ulnar nerve transposed anteriorly and fascial flap sutured to anterior subcutaneous tissue.

SUMMARY

Pitchers are prone to elbow injuries because of high and repetitive valgus stresses on the elbow. The anterior bundle of the MCL of the elbow is the primary restraint and often attenuated with time, leading to functional incompetence and ultimate failure. Pitchers with a history of medial elbow pain, reduced velocity, and loss of command may have an MCL injury in evolution. Physical examination and imaging can confirm the diagnosis. Treatment begins with rest and activity modification. All medial elbow pain is not MCL injury. Surgery is considered only for talented athletes who wish to return to competitive play and may include elite scholastic and other collegiates and professionals. Since Jobe and colleagues[3] first described their technique for MCL reconstruction in 1986, variations have been offered, which can result in predictable outcomes, allowing many to return to the same level of competitive play.

REFERENCES

1. Bennet G. Shoulder and elbow lesions of the professional baseball pitcher. JAMA 1941;117:510–4.
2. Waris W. Elbow injuries in javelin throwers. Acta Chir Scand 1946;93:563–75.
3. Jobe FW, Stark H, Lombardo SJ. Reconstruction of the ulnar collateral ligament in athletes. J Bone Joint Surg Am 1986;68(8):1158–63.
4. Schwab GH, Bennett JB, Woods GW, et al. Biomechanics of elbow instability: the role of the medial collateral ligament. Clin Orthop Relat Res 1980; 146:42–52.
5. Morrey BF. Applied anatomy and biomechanics of the elbow joint. Instr Course Lect 1986;35:59–68.
6. Regan WD, Korinek SL, Morrey BF, et al. Biomechanical study of ligaments around the elbow joint. Clin Orthop Relat Res 1991;271:170–9.
7. Callaway GH, Field LD, Deng XH, et al. Biomechanical evaluation of the medial collateral ligament of the elbow. J Bone Joint Surg Am 1997;79(8):1223–31.
8. Jobe F, Kvitne R. Elbow instability in the athlete. Instr Course Lect 1991;40:17–23.
9. Pappas AM, Zawacki RM, Sullivan TJ. Biomechanics of baseball pitching. A preliminary report. Am J Sports Med 1985;13(4):216–22.
10. Fleisig GS, Barrentine SW, Zheng N, et al. Kinematic and kinetic comparison of baseball pitching among various levels of development. J Biomech 1999; 32(12):1371–5.
11. Ahmad CS, Lee TQ, ElAttrache NS. Biomechanical evaluation of a new ulnar collateral ligament reconstruction technique with interference screw fixation. Am J Sports Med 2003;31(3):332–7.
12. Morrey BF, An KN. Articular and ligamentous contributions to the stability of the elbow joint. Am J Sports Med 1983;11(5):315–9.
13. Lynch JR, Waitayawinyu T, Hanel DP, et al. Medial collateral ligament injury in the overhand-throwing athlete. J Hand Surg [Am] 2008;33(3):430–7.
14. Conway JE, Jobe FW, Glousman RE, et al. Medial instability of the elbow in throwing athletes. Treatment by repair or reconstruction of the ulnar collateral ligament. J Bone Joint Surg Am 1992;74(1):67–83.
15. O'Driscoll SW, Lawton RL, Smith AM. The "moving valgus stress test" for medial collateral ligament tears of the elbow. Am J Sports Med 2005;33(2): 231–9.
16. Sasaki J, Takahara M, Ogino T, et al. Ultrasonographic assessment of the ulnar collateral ligament and medial elbow laxity in college baseball players. J Bone Joint Surg Am 2002;84-A(4):525–31.
17. Mirowitz SA, London SL. Ulnar collateral ligament injury in baseball pitchers: MR imaging evaluation. Radiology 1992;185(2):573–6.
18. Hill NB Jr, Bucchieri JS, Shon F, et al. Magnetic resonance imaging of injury to the medial collateral ligament of the elbow: a cadaver model. J Shoulder Elbow Surg 2000;9(5):418–22.
19. Schwartz ML, al-Zahrani S, Morwessel RM, et al. Ulnar collateral ligament injury in the throwing athlete: evaluation with saline-enhanced MR arthrography. Radiology 1995;197(1):297–9.
20. Rettig AC, Sherrill C, Snead DS, et al. Nonoperative treatment of ulnar collateral ligament injuries in throwing athletes. Am J Sports Med 2001;29(1):15–7.
21. Smith GR, Altchek DW, Pagnani MJ, et al. A muscle-splitting approach to the ulnar collateral ligament of the elbow. Neuroanatomy and operative technique. Am J Sports Med 1996;24(5):575–80.
22. Rohrbough JT, Altchek DW, Hyman J, et al. Medial collateral ligament reconstruction of the elbow using

the docking technique. Am J Sports Med 2002; 30(4):541–8.

23. Vitale MA, Ahmad CS. The outcome of elbow ulnar collateral ligament reconstruction in overhead athletes: a systematic review. Am J Sports Med 2008;36(6):1193–205.

24. Paletta GA Jr, Wright RW. The modified docking procedure for elbow ulnar collateral ligament reconstruction: 2-year follow-up in elite throwers. Am J Sports Med 2006;34(10):1594–8.

25. Koh JL, Schafer MF, Keuter G, et al. Ulnar collateral ligament reconstruction in elite throwing athletes. Arthroscopy 2006;22(11):1187–91.

26. Arendt E. OKU orthopaedic knowledge update. Sports medicine 2. Rosemont, IL: AAOS; 1999. 225–235.

Biceps Tendon Injuries in Athletes

Zinon T. Kokkalis, MD, Dean G. Sotereanos, MD*

KEYWORDS

- Distal biceps tendon • Injuries • Athletes • Elbow
- Repair • Reconstruction

Athletes involved in strength training and contact sports such as competitive weightlifting, professional bodybuilding, football, and rugby may sustain distal biceps tendon injuries. Even though causes of these injuries are still portrayed as controversial and multifactorial in etiology, the mechanism of injury is still perceived as a single traumatic event involving forceful eccentric contraction of the muscle. Use of anabolic steroids in power lifters may predispose to these lesions. Early surgical intervention with anatomic reattachment of the ruptured tendon to the bicipital tuberosity is recommended. The ideal repair technique should be one that provides anatomic repair with high fixation strength, so as to obtain early motion, with an extremely low complication rate. This article focuses on all significant types of biceps tendon injuries in athletes by identifying its diagnostic modalities and surgical indications as well as all aspects of their treatment options, surgical techniques, and potential complications.

SURGICAL ANATOMY

Thorough knowledge of the anatomy of the distal biceps tendon may assist surgeons in correctly orientating the distal biceps tendon during anatomic repair, thus restoring more normal muscle kinematics.[1] The biceps brachii is a long spindle-shaped muscle, placed in the anterior compartment of the arm. It arises by the short and long heads, which merge at the level of the deltoid tuberosity to form a single muscle belly. This muscle belly ends in a flattened tendon, which passes deep in the antecubital fossa to insert into the bicipital tuberosity on the proximal radius.[2,3] The distal biceps tendon inserts on the ulnar aspect of the tuberosity as a ribbon-shaped insertion footprint.[4–6] Anatomic descriptions showed that the long head of the distal tendon inserts onto the proximal aspect of the bicipital tuberosity, whereas the short head of the distal tendon inserts onto the distal aspect of the tuberosity.[1,7] On average, the biceps tendon insertion starts 23 mm distal to the articular margin of the radial head, and the average total area of the biceps tendon insertion (footprint) is 108 mm^2.[1] A bursa interposes between the distal biceps tendon and the front part of the tuberosity. At the junction of the musculotendinous unit and the distal biceps tendon, the lacertus fibrosus or bicipital aponeurosis arises from the medial side of the muscle belly and passes obliquely in an ulnar direction, merging with the fascia covering the proximal flexor mass of the forearm.[2,3,7–9]

During surgery, the surgeon should be aware of the various neurovascular structures that course into the antecubital fossa.[9,10] The antecubital fossa is the triangular area which is formed between the pronator teres medially and the brachioradialis laterally. The floor of the fossa is formed by the brachialis and by the supinator laterally. It contains the biceps tendon, brachial artery, and median nerve, from lateral to medial. The brachial artery usually bifurcates at the apex of the antecubital fossa into the radial and ulnar arteries. Close to its origin, the radial artery gives off the recurrent radial artery, which traverses

No declared financial interests for both authors in any form have been received or will be received from a commercial party related directly or indirectly to the subject of this article.

Department of Orthopaedic Surgery, Hand and Upper Extremity Surgery, Allegheny General Hospital, 1307 Federal Street, 2nd Floor, Pittsburgh, PA 15212, USA

* Corresponding author.

E-mail address: dsoterea@hotmail.com (D.G. Sotereanos).

doi:10.1016/j.hcl.2009.05.007

hand.theclinics.com

laterally and proximally across the antecubital fossa. The biceps brachii receives innervation by way of the musculocutaneous nerve (C5, C6) from the lateral cord of the brachial plexus. Its terminal branch, the lateral antebrachial cutaneous nerve, descends lateral to the biceps tendon into the superficial fascia and it is vulnerable to iatrogenic injury.[11–13] The radial nerve pierces the lateral intermuscular septum, and courses between the brachialis and brachioradialis to the front of the lateral epicondyle, where it divides into a superficial and a deep branch. The superficial branch continues into the forearm beneath the brachioradialis and lateral to the radial artery. The deep branch (posterior interosseous nerve) courses around the lateral neck of the radius and enters between the two planes of fibers of the supinator, where it can be at risk for injury during surgery.[12–17]

BIOMECHANICS

The biceps brachii is the most powerful supinator of the forearm, and serves elbow flexion in conjunction with the brachialis muscle. Eames and colleagues,[7] in a cadaveric study, showed that the short head, inserted distal to the radial tuberosity, is a more powerful flexor of the elbow, whereas the tendon of the long head, inserted on the tuberosity further from the axis of rotation of the forearm, is a stronger supinator. These functions of the biceps are influenced by the position of the forearm. It is well known that the biceps muscle becomes less active on the prone forearm. The flexor function is augmented when the forearm is in a supinated position, and the biceps becomes the primary supinator of the forearm with progressive flexion of the elbow at 90°.[18,19]

PATHOPHYSIOLOGY

Distal biceps tendon rupture was encountered rarely as an injury; only 65 cases were reported before 1941.[4,20] However, Safran and Graham[21] recently reported an increased frequency in incidences of 1.2 ruptures per 100,000 persons per year. In the average population, the rupture typically occurs in the dominant extremity of active males between the fourth and sixth decades of life, although recent literature has shown that individuals of any age and of either gender can be affected.[9,11,17,22–28] In athletes, these injuries do occur in younger age groups.[23,29,30] Distal biceps injury is rare in the overhead athletes but it is more common in weight lifters and bodybuilders.[23,29]

The mechanism of distal biceps injury has been reported as the result of forceful eccentric contraction of the muscle.[31] During a single traumatic event, a sudden extension force is applied to a flexed, supinated forearm resulting in rupture of the distal biceps.[9,20–24,32–35] The tendon typically avulses from the radial tuberosity, whereas the bicipital aponeurosis may or may not rupture. An intact bicipital aponeurosis prevents proximal migration of the ruptured tendon into the arm.

A variety of degenerative, hypovascular, and mechanical factors contribute or even finally cause the tendon tear.[21,23,30,36–38] Spontaneous rupture of a tendon, almost without exception, is preceded by degenerative changes–degenerative or calcifying tendinopathy or mucoid degeneration.[37] Seiler and colleagues[36] described the interaction of mechanical impingement on the biceps tendon during forearm rotation and hypovascularity as a potential cause. They identified three vascular zones in the distal biceps tendon and reported that a hypovascular zone, averaging 2.14 cm, was evident between the proximal and distal zones. The same group found that the cross-sectional area through the proximal radioulnar joint at the radial tuberosity decreased almost 50% from full supination to full pronation. Eames and colleagues,[7] reported that increased tension of the lacertus fibrosus during strong forearm rotation may contribute to additional mechanical impingement. Other reports suggest that a prominent edge of the bicipital tuberosity erodes the tendon during pronation, rendering it vulnerable to rupture when exposed to high forces.[4,39] This may be analogous to subacromial impingement and rotator cuff tears.

Abuse of anabolic steroids and nicotine are factors discussed in the literature as being possibly related to distal biceps degeneration and rupture.[21,40–42] Bodybuilders commonly abuse a variety of steroids, such as testosterone and nandrolone. Often, several different androgens are used over prolonged periods of time in doses far in excess of normal levels to achieve the desired effect.[42] Muscular strength is increased, but the tendon becomes stiffer and absorbs less energy, so it is more likely to fail during competitive sport activities.[40] However, in the only series looking specifically at this injury in athletes, most of whom were weight lifters (8 out of 10), all the patients denied steroid use.[23]

CLASSIFICATION

Distal biceps tendon ruptures can be categorized as partial or complete. Partial ruptures are rare and often triggered by minor trauma without even being associated with a traumatic incident. Preexisting degeneration in the tendon is accounted by the latter situation.[8] A subdivision of partial ruptures into insertional (to bone) and intra-substance (tendon elongation), as seen on the MRI, was described by Ramsey.[9]

Complete ruptures are arbitrarily classified as acute and chronic, based on the time period between injury and diagnosis. Biceps ruptures occurring within 4 weeks are considered acute, and an anatomic repair is feasible.[33–35] Injuries presenting after 4 weeks are classified as chronic and are further subdivided based on the integrity of the lacertus fibrosus. The importance of defining the chronicity of the rupture and the integrity of the lacertus fibrosus lies in its usefulness in predicting the ease of repair and the anticipated outcome.[9] In cases of a torn lacertus with proximal retraction of the biceps tendon, direct reattachment of the biceps may be difficult, if not impossible, making the procedure more challenging.[33,43–45]

DIAGNOSIS
Clinical Examination

Diagnosis of the distal biceps rupture is mainly established on the basis of history, mechanism of injury, and clinical examination. Patients with complete distal biceps rupture usually report a traumatic event where an unexpected extension force was applied to the flexed arm, although others report that they attempted to avoid a sudden fall.[46] This is usually associated with an audible pop or a snapping sensation followed by pain and weakness in the upper extremity. The intense pain often recedes in a few hours, and is followed by a dull aching pain which can last for weeks to months.[32] On physical examination, swelling and ecchymosis in the antecubital fossa extending distally and proximally are usually seen in the acute phase. A defect in the antecubital fossa can be palpated, and proximal migration of the biceps muscle belly can be seen with active elbow flexion. Most patients, especially body builders, appreciate a difference in the appearance in the arm.[23] If the bicipital aponeurosis is intact, the deformity is not as marked. Differential diagnosis should include rupture of the long head of the biceps at the tendon-labrum junction which gives the classic Popeye appearance of the biceps (distal retraction of the muscle belly) (**Fig. 1**).

Atypical presentations, and partial or subacute and/or chronic injuries, may lack some or all of the above findings and create a diagnostic dilemma. In cases of partial distal biceps rupture, pain to palpation in the antecubital fossa with resisted supination is the most common finding.

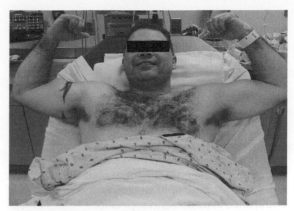

Fig. 1. Classic Popeye appearance of the biceps muscle after rupture of the long head of the biceps at the tendon-labrum junction (distal retraction of the muscle belly of the right biceps).

Active flexion and supination strength are usually limited by pain.[27] Patients with chronic distal biceps ruptures usually present late after a discrete traumatic event with dull pain and weakness in elbow flexion and forearm supination. Asymmetry in the contour of the muscle and dysesthesias in the lateral antebrachial cutaneous nerve distribution may be noted.[43,44]

Moreover, the "biceps squeeze" test[47] and the "hook" test,[48] whose specificity and sensitivity were reported as very high, might be helpful tests for diagnosing distal biceps tendon avulsions, whether acute or chronic.

Radiographic Studies

The diagnosis of a distal biceps tendon rupture can be made clinically for most patients. However, in difficult cases paraclinical studies are warranted. Plain radiographs can occasionally reveal enlargement or irregularity of the radial tuberosity,[4,39] as well as avulsion of a part of the bicipital tuberosity. Ultrasonography or MRI may provide useful information on cases with partial tear or ruptures that are not retracted because of an intact aponeurosis.[49–51] Although MRI is the gold standard for the imaging evaluation of the elbow, sonography is less expensive and more rapidly performed, and the contralateral normal elbow is readily available for comparison.[49] MRI findings associated with a partial tear commonly include the presence of increased intratendinous signal and an abnormal tendon diameter. Bicipital bursitis, peritendinous fluid, and marrow edema at the biceps insertion may also be evident.[8,51,52] An innovative MRI technique of positioning the patient with the shoulder abducted, elbow flexed, and forearm supinated (FABS position) was recently described.[52] This view can complement conventional MRI in cases in which other pathologic conditions are implicated, such as tenosynovitis, tendinitis, or bursitis.[8,52]

SURGICAL INDICATIONS

Treatment of complete distal biceps tendon ruptures in athletes is primarily surgical. Nonoperative management was the mainstay of treatment for distal biceps ruptures in the past.[53,54] Nevertheless, conservative treatment of distal biceps tears led to an appreciable decrease in strength and endurance in flexion and supination.[24,33,55] Nonoperative treatment showed a 40% loss of supination strength and an average 30% loss of flexion strength.[33] Pearl and colleagues[56] reported on a weight lifter's strength deficits after biceps tendon rupture and the advantages of surgical repair over nonoperative treatment, since both treatment options had been employed in the same patient. In this case the unrepaired biceps tendon showed 48% less supination strength and 39% less flexion strength than the repaired side.

Acute surgical repair with anatomic reinsertion of the ruptured tendon to the bicipital tuberosity is favored in active individuals of all ages, athletes as well as non-athletes.[9-11,23-30,33-35,46,55-59] Early repair (within 2 weeks) is clearly the treatment of choice in athletes, although good results have been reported with delayed reconstruction.[23] In a poll of National Football League team physicians, 90% favored early repair of distal biceps ruptures during the season games, rather than postponing surgery until the end of the season.[60]

Anatomic reattachment with or without autograft and/or allograft should be attempted in active individuals with chronic injuries.[44,51,55,57,58] Nonanatomic attachment (transfer) of the biceps tendon to the brachialis muscle is favored by some surgeons so as to avoid any potential complications associated with deep surgical dissection and the use of the graft; even though supination strength is not restored.[35,61,62] In this situation, the significant loss of supination strength may be unacceptable for patients with high functional requirements in supination, such as manual workers and athletes, and it must be discussed with them before surgery.

SURGICAL TREATMENT
Complete Ruptures

The goal of any surgical procedure to repair the distal biceps tendon rupture should be restoration of the pre-injury anatomy and function as closely as possible. Single-incision and two-incision

techniques, with various modifications, have been extensively described, each having its advantages and limitations. Controversy still exists over which approach is superior.

In 1961, Boyd and Anderson[63] were the first to introduce the two-incision technique in an effort to limit surgical dissection and prevent neurologic injury. This technique involves a small anterior incision and a second posterolateral incision. However, an increased incidence of proximal radioulnar synostosis was related with their technique.[33,64]

Failla and colleagues[64] postulated that the development of synostosis was related to proximal interosseous membrane damage and stimulation of the ulnar periosteum because of subperiosteal exposure of the ulna. They prompted for a modified two-incision technique in which a limited muscle-splitting approach through the extensor muscle mass was used; thus, subperiosteal exposure of the ulna is avoided. They also recommended copious wound irrigation to remove bone dust produced from the use of a burr to create a trough in the radial tuberosity. Although this tailored approach theoretically decreases the risk for radioulnar synostosis and heterotopic ossification, the possibility of synostosis has not been eliminated.[13,58,65,66]

In the past, anatomic repair was performed through an extensile single anterior approach with sutures to bone, resulting in an increased incidence of nerve injuries.[20,54] With the introduction of newer fixation devices such as bone suture anchors, EndoButton (Acufex, Smith & Nephew, Andover, Massachusetts), and interference Biotenodesis screws (Arthrex, Naples, Florida), a single-incision anterior approach without extensive dissection of the proximal radius has become increasingly more popular.[17,27,46,67-73]

Authors' Preferred Technique

The authors favor distal biceps repair through a single anterior approach with suture anchor technique.[27,43,46] Surgery is performed under general or regional anesthesia, with the patient in supine position and the affected arm on a hand table. The procedure is performed using an arm tourniquet, preset to 250 mm Hg. A single, S-shaped, anterior incision is centered over the antecubital fossa, facilitating a modified Henry's approach (**Fig. 2**). The lateral antebrachial cutaneous nerve is identified and retracted laterally. The deep fascia is incised, and the distal biceps tendon is identified. If the lacertus fibrosus is intact, the tendon will remain in the tendon sheath. If the lacertus fibrosus is ruptured, the tendon will

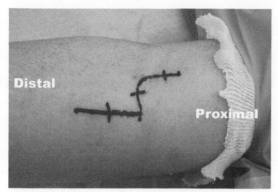

Fig. 2. A single, modified, anterior Henry incision, centered over the antecubital fossa, is used for the procedure.

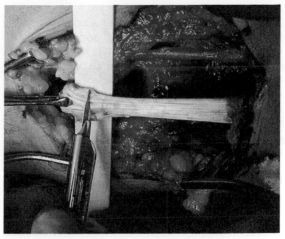

Fig. 4. The tendon is adequately debrided, approximately 5–10 mm, to normal tendon substance.

retract proximally into the anterior compartment of the arm. In chronic cases, the tendon may be enclosed in a cocoon of connective tissue that might give the impression of tendon continuity to the bicipital tuberosity (**Fig. 3**). The tendon sheath is incised longitudinally, and the tendon is retrieved and adequately debrided, approximately 5 to 10 mm, to normal tendon substance (**Fig. 4**). The interval between the brachioradialis and pronator teres is identified and dissected, and right angle retractors are placed between these muscles. The radial recurrent vessels are ligated to facilitate retraction, which allows safe distal exposure of the bicipital tuberosity. The radial attachment of the supinator is not released. The radial nerve and posterior interosseous nerve are not exposed; instead, they are protected by gentle retraction and, most important, by keeping the forearm fully

supinated. The bicipital tuberosity is exposed and cleared of soft tissue, including residual tendon stump, with a small periosteal elevator.

Two anchors (Mitek GII, DePuy Mitek, Norwood, Massachusetts), loaded with No. 2 nonabsorbable sutures, are placed in parallel and approximately 1 cm apart into the bicipital tuberosity. The two sutures attached to the anchors are independently passed trough the distal 3 cm of the tendon with a sliding Kessler stitch,[27] and then tied securely through the biceps footprint (**Fig. 5**). The elbow is maintained in full supination and approximately 60° of elbow flexion during suture tying. Routine closure of the wound is then completed. The arm is placed in a well padded posterior splint with the elbow in 90° of flexion and the forearm in 20° of supination.

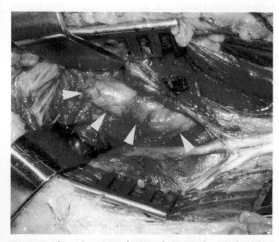

Fig. 3. In chronic cases, the tendon may be enclosed in a cocoon of connective tissue (*arrows*) that might give the impression of tendon continuity to the bicipital tuberosity.

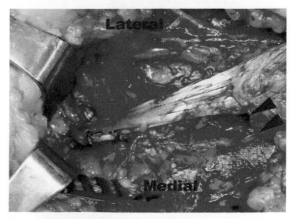

Fig. 5. Using a modified Kessler sliding stitch the distal biceps tendon is repaired to the bicipital tuberosity. In this case of acute complete distal biceps rupture, the lacertus fibrosus was disrupted (*arrowheads*).

Postoperative regimen

A dynamic, hinged extension block brace is applied at the first postoperative visit, approximately 10 days postoperatively, in 45° of extension (**Fig. 6**). This dynamic brace uses elastic bands to allow active assisted elbow flexion. It is kept in place to protect the repair for 6 to 8 weeks. The brace is adjusted weekly and range of motion is advanced to full extension progressively starting at the third week. Active motion is permitted after 6 weeks, and resisted supination and flexion are not allowed for 12 weeks after surgery. Strengthening exercises begin at the fourth month and unrestricted activities are typically allowed at 4 to 6 months.[27,43,46]

Chronic Ruptures

Chronic distal biceps ruptures are more difficult to repair and the outcomes of late reconstruction are considered inferior and less predictable than those of acute repair.[33,43–45,57–59,62,74–77] Biceps muscle retraction, distal tendon shortening, and adhesion formation are common drawbacks when attempting to repair chronic ruptures (usually more than 6 weeks after injury). In such cases, the surgeon has three options: to attempt to mobilize the biceps and perform an anatomic repair, to perform a nonanatomic repair (transfer) of the distal biceps to the brachialis muscle, or to perform distal biceps tendon reconstruction. Distal biceps mobilization can be achieved by sectioning the lacertus fibrosus (if it is intact), releasing adhesions, performing relaxing incisions to the epimysium, and applying

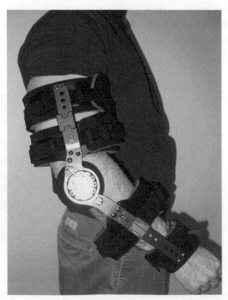

Fig. 6. A dynamic, hinged extension block brace is applied at the first postoperative visit, in 45° of extension.

traction to the distal biceps stump for several minutes.[43,46] These measures, although helpful, are seldom effective. Tenodesis of the retracted tendon to the distal brachialis muscle is the simpler salvage procedure and may increase elbow flexion strength; however, this procedure does not restore supination strength and endurance.[33,35,61,62]

Autograft options for late reconstruction of retracted chronic ruptures include fascia lata,[75,76] semitendinosus,[44,45] and flexor carpi radialis.[59,77] Achilles tendon allograft has also been advocated[43,74] and can be used if the patient wishes to avoid donor-site morbidity. Late reconstruction through a single anterior approach using Achilles tendon allograft is the authors' preferred technique. Although this technique is a demanding procedure and involves a prolonged rehabilitation period, it is an excellent alternative for patients with high functional demands in pronosupination, such as athletes. Although no major complications were encountered in the authors' series,[43] the possibility of infection and remote disease transmission from the allograft must be taken into consideration and discussed with the patient before the surgery.

Partial Ruptures

Partial distal biceps tendon ruptures are atypical, and in the professional athlete, an MRI is probably desirable to confirm the diagnosis. These ruptures are initially treated conservatively with nonsteroidal antiinflammatory drugs, splinting, and physiotherapy. These measures may lead occasionally to complete recovery.[78] Surgical treatment is reserved only for refractory cases.[11,26–28,79] Surgical excision of degenerative tendon, either through a single- or two-incision technique, debridement of the frayed tendon end, and anatomic reinsertion to the radial tuberosity are recommended.[26–28,79]

From their series,[27] the authors reported on seven patients who underwent surgical debridement and reattachment of the biceps tendon using a single-incision technique with suture anchors. Intraoperatively, in all cases the tendon had significant degeneration and softening at the insertion site, but it was in partial continuity with the radial tuberosity. Approximately 1 cm of the degenerated portion of the tendon was excised to normal tendon fibers, and anatomic repair was performed. Postoperatively, there was a significant decrease in pain, and flexion and supination strengths were comparable to those in the contralateral arm.[27] Dellaero and Mallon[11] also reported successful outcomes from using the same technique (completion of the tear and reattachment through a single incision with suture anchors).

RESULTS

It is well documented in recent literature that early anatomic reattachment of the tendon to the biceps tuberosity in acute and subacute injuries will result in return to elbow flexion and supination strength and endurance.[9–11,23–28,33–35,46,55–59,67–73] The ideal distal biceps tendon repair should have high fixation strength, allow early rehabilitation, and have extremely low complication rate. As mentioned, single-incision and two-incision techniques, with various modifications, have evolved over time. Many clinical reports found no difference in the functional outcomes between these two techniques.[57,80,81] The decision between a one- or two-incision technique depends on the surgeon's preference and experience level.[10]

D'Alessandro and colleagues,[23] in the only published series with distal biceps tendon ruptures in athletes, performed a modified two-incision technique for all of their patients, which were predominantly weight lifters and body builders. They reported that all athletes were satisfied with the cosmetic appearance and returned to full, unrestricted activity. Other surgeons report that using this technique, early range of motion may be instituted with excellent results.[32–34,55,60] Complications associated with this procedure are proximal radioulnar synostosis and heterotopic ossification.[12,13,23,55,58] This limited single anterior exposure theoretically diminishes the risk for radioulnar synostosis and heterotopic ossification associated with a dorsal incision. However, bone quality needs to be considered, since many of the newer generation suture anchors require and depend on anterior cortical bone of the bicipital tuberosity for fixation.[70] Additionally, if the biceps tendon is not repaired to its anatomic position and is merely inserted into the center of the bicipital tuberosity, the power of supination may never be restored to pre-injury levels.[5]

Recent biomechanical studies have compared the various fixation techniques. The results are conflicting. Pereira and colleagues[82] reported that the two-incision bone-tunnel technique of distal biceps repair was found to have significantly greater yield force and force to failure in the group of younger, nonosteoporotic elbows than the one-incision suture anchor technique. Conversely, Lemos and colleagues,[83] using a newer suture anchor fixation technique, found this repair an equal if not superior alternative to bone tunnel fixation in the specimens tested. Other studies reported that the interference screw provides better stiffness and failure strength compared with the bone tunnel technique[84] or suture anchors.[85] Spang and colleagues[86] found comparable fixation strength for the repair and rehabilitation when compared to suture anchor and EndoButton repair in a human bone-tendon model. On the other hand, Mazzocca and colleagues[87] performed a comparative biomechanical analysis of four distal biceps tendon repair techniques: transosseous bone tunnel fixation (two-incision technique), suture anchor repair, EndoButton, and interference screw fixation. These authors concluded that the EndoButton technique provided the highest load to failure when compared with each of the other techniques.

COMPLICATIONS

The main complication of the original single-incision technique has been neurologic sequelae. Lateral antebrachial cutaneous nerve paresthesia and subsequent posterior interosseous nerve palsy were the most common nerve injuries.[14,15,17,20,57] With the introduction of newer fixation devices, the anterior one-incision technique was made feasible by limiting extensive soft-tissue dissection, resulting in minimal morbidity and a low complication rate. McKee and colleagues,[17] in a series of 53 patients, reported only 3 (5.6%) neurologic complications and an overall complication rate of 7.5% (4/53) for all patients who were treated with an anterior one-incision technique with suture anchors. Ectopic bone formation is rare after one-insicion technique. However, the authors had to revise two cases that were previously repaired with EndoButton technique and developed ectopic bone formation (**Fig. 7**).

The major complications with the two-incision technique are radioulnar synostosis and heterotopic ossification.[12,13,58,63–66] Nerve injuries have also been described in literature.[12,13,16] Synostosis formation is attributed to aggressive subperiosteal release of the anconeus muscle from the ulna.[34] Early resection of the synostosis, if it develops, is the only treatment to restore a functional range of forearm rotation, but the results are unpredictable.[65,66] Kelly and colleagues[12] reported the complications of the two-incision technique using the muscle-splitting modification. In their study of 74 repairs, six patients (8.1%) developed nerve injuries, which included five sensory nerve paresthesias and one temporary palsy of the posterior interosseous nerve. There were no cases of radioulnar synostosis, but four patients developed heterotopic ossification. On the contrary, Bisson and colleagues,[13] using the same modified two-incision technique in 45 patients, reported functional radioulnar synostosis in three patients (7%) and loss of forearm rotation unrelated to

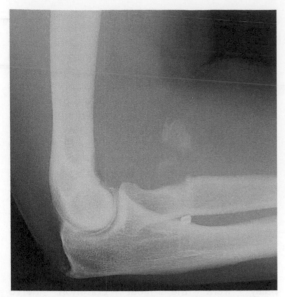

Fig. 7. In this patient, ectopic bone formation along the distal biceps tendon repaired with EndoButton technique is clearly shown. He was a body builder who presented with pain and functional limitation 4 months after surgery.

heterotopic ossification in two patients. There was an overall complication rate of 27%.

Finally, rerupture is an exceptionally rare complication with any method of biceps repair, even when, anecdotally, patients do not adhere to their postoperative rehabilitation restrictions.[88]

SUMMARY

Distal biceps injuries are rare in overhead athletes, but they are more common in weight lifters and bodybuilders. The etiology and pathophysiology of tendon ruptures is controversial and multifactorial. Treatment of complete distal biceps tendon tears in athletes is primarily surgical, as this is the best method to restore both flexion and supination strength and endurance. Surgical repair, through either one-incision or two-incision technique, with anatomic reinsertion of the ruptured tendon to the bicipital tuberosity, is highly recommended. Selection of the technique should be based on surgeon preference, surgeon training, and comfort level with the approaches. Early surgical repair (within 2 weeks) will usually yield excellent results.

REFERENCES

1. Athwal GS, Steinmann SP, Rispoli DM. The distal biceps tendon: footprint and relevant clinical anatomy. J Hand Surg [Am] 2007;32(8):1225–9.

2. Koch S, Tillmann B. The distal tendon of the biceps brachii. Structure and clinical correlations. Ann Anat 1995;177(5):467–74.

3. Standring S. Gray's anatomy: the anatomical basis of clinical practice. 39th edition. Edinburgh, Scotland: Elsevier Churchill Livingstone; 2005. p. 853.

4. Mazzocca AD, Cohen M, Berkson E, et al. The anatomy of the bicipital tuberosity and distal biceps tendon. J Shoulder Elbow Surg 2007;16(1):122–7.

5. Hutchinson HL, Gloystein D, Gillespie M. Distal biceps tendon insertion: an anatomic study. J Shoulder Elbow Surg 2008;17(2):342–6.

6. Forthman CL, Zimmerman RM, Sullivan MJ, et al. Cross-sectional anatomy of the bicipital tuberosity and biceps brachii tendon insertion: relevance to anatomic tendon repair. J Shoulder Elbow Surg 2008;17:522–6.

7. Eames MH, Bain GI, Fogg QA, et al. Distal biceps tendon anatomy: a cadaveric study. J Bone Joint Surg Am 2007;89(5):1044–9.

8. Chew ML, Giuffrè BM. Disorders of the distal biceps brachii tendon. Radiographics 2005;25(5): 1227–37.

9. Ramsey ML. Distal biceps tendon injuries: diagnosis and management. J Am Acad Orthop Surg 1999; 7(3):199–207.

10. Vidal AF, Drakos MC, Allen AA. Biceps tendon and triceps tendon injuries. Clin Sports Med 2004; 23(4):707–22.

11. Dellaero DT, Mallon WJ. Surgical treatment of partial biceps tendon ruptures at the elbow. J Shoulder Elbow Surg 2006;15(2):215–7.

12. Kelly EW, Morrey BF, O'Driscoll SW. Complications of repair of the distal biceps tendon with the modified 2-incision technique. J Bone Joint Surg Am 2000;82:1575–81.

13. Bisson L, Moyer M, Lanighan K, et al. Complications associated with repair of a distal biceps rupture using the modified 2-incision technique. J Shoulder Elbow Surg 2008;17:67S–71S.

14. Saldua N, Carney J, Dewing C, et al. The effect of drilling angle on posterior interosseous nerve safety during open and endoscopic anterior single-incision repair of the distal biceps tendon. Arthroscopy 2008;24(3):305–10.

15. Katzman BM, Caligiuri DA, Klein DM, et al. Delayed onset of posterior interosseous nerve palsy after distal biceps tendon repair. J Shoulder Elbow Surg 1997;6(4):393–5.

16. Stearns KL, Sarris I, Sotereanos DG. Permanent posterior interosseous nerve palsy following a 2-incision distal biceps tendon repair. Orthopedics 2004; 27(8):867–8.

17. McKee MD, Hirji R, Schemitsch EH, et al. Patient-oriented functional outcome after repair of distal biceps tendon ruptures using a single-incision technique. J Shoulder Elbow Surg 2005;14(3):302–6.

18. Naito A, Shimizu Y, Handa Y, et al. Functional anatomical studies of the elbow movements. I. Electromyographic (EMG) analysis. Okajimas Folia Anat Jpn 1991;68(5):283–8.

19. Basmajian JV, Latif MA. Integrated actions and functions of the chief flexors of the elbow. J Bone Joint Surg Am 1957;39:1106–18.

20. Dobbie RP. Avulsion of the lower biceps brachii tendon. Analysis of 51 previously unreported cases. Am J Surg 1941;51:662–3.

21. Safran MR, Graham SM. Distal biceps tendon ruptures: incidence, demographics, and the effect of smoking. Clin Orthop 2002;404:275–83.

22. Boucher PR, Morton KS. Rupture of the distal biceps brachii tendon. J Trauma 1967;7(5):626–32.

23. D'Alessandro DF, Shields CL Jr, Tibone JE, et al. Repair of distal biceps tendon ruptures in athletes. Am J Sports Med 1993;21(1):114–9.

24. Leighton MM, Bush-Joseph CA, Bach BR Jr. Distal biceps brachii repair. Results in dominant and nondominant extremities. Clin Orthop Relat Res 1995;(317):114–21.

25. Toczylowski HM, Balint CR, Steiner ME, et al. Complete rupture of the distal biceps brachii tendon in female patients: a report of 2 cases. J Shoulder Elbow Surg 2002;11:516–8.

26. Rokito AS, McLaughlin JA, Gallagher MA, et al. Partial rupture of the distal biceps tendon. J Shoulder Elbow Surg 1996;5:73–5.

27. Vardakas DG, Musgrave DS, Varitimidis SE, et al. Partial rupture of the distal biceps tendon. J Shoulder Elbow Surg 2001;10:377–9.

28. Bourne MH, Morrey BF. Partial rupture of the distal biceps tendon. Clin Orthop 1991;271:143–8.

29. Alberta FG, Elattrache NS. Diagnosis and treatment of distal biceps and anterior elbow pain in throwing athletes. Sports Med Arthrosc 2008; 16(3):118–23.

30. Kannus P, Natri A. Etiology and pathophysiology of tendon ruptures in sports. Scand J Med Sci Sports 1997;7(2):107–12.

31. Acquaviva P. Rupture du tendon inferieur du biceps brachial droit a son insertion sur la tuberosite bicipitale: tenosuture succes operatoire. Mars Med 1898;35: 570–3 [in French].

32. Morrey BF. Tendon injuries about the elbow. In: Morrey BF, editor. The elbow and its disorders. Philadelphia: WB Saunders; 1993. p. 492–504.

33. Morrey BF, Askew LJ, An KN, et al. Rupture of distal tendon of the biceps brachii: a biomechanical study. J Bone Joint Surg 1985;67:418–21.

34. D'Arco P, Sitler M, Kelly J, et al. Clinical, functional, and radiographic assessments of the conventional and modified Boyd-Anderson surgical procedures for repair of distal biceps tendon ruptures. Am J Sports Med 1998;26:254–61.

35. Bell RH, Wiley WB, Noble JS, et al. Repair of distal biceps brachii tendon ruptures. J Shoulder Elbow Surg 2000;9(3):223–6.

36. Seiler JG III, Parker LM, Chamberland PD, et al. The distal biceps tendon: two potential mechanisms involved in its rupture-arterial supply and mechanical impingement. J Shoulder Elbow Surg 1995;4:149–56.

37. Kannus P, Józsa L. Histopathological changes preceding spontaneous rupture of a tendon. A controlled study of 891 patients. J Bone Joint Surg Am 1991;73(10):1507–25.

38. Kulshreshtha R, Singh R, Sinha J, et al. Anatomy of the distal biceps brachii tendon and its clinical relevance. Clin Orthop Relat Res 2007;456:117–20.

39. Davis WM, Yassine Z. An etiological factor in tear of the distal tendon of the biceps brachii. Report of 2 cases. J Bone Joint Surg Am 1956;38:1365–8.

40. Miles JW, Grana WA, Egle D, et al. The effect of anabolic steroids on the biomechanical and histological properties of rat tendon. J Bone Joint Surg Am 1992;74(3):411–22.

41. Visuri T, Lindholm H. Bilateral distal biceps tendon avulsions with use of anabolic steroids. Med Sci Sports Exerc 1994;26(8):941–4.

42. Cope MR, Ali A, Bayliss NC. Biceps rupture in body builders: three case reports of rupture of the long head of the biceps at the tendon-labrum junction. J Shoulder Elbow Surg 2004;13(5):580–2.

43. Darlis NA, Sotereanos DG. Distal biceps tendon reconstruction in chronic ruptures. J Shoulder Elbow Surg 2006;15(5):614–9.

44. Hang DW, Bach BR Jr, Bojchuk J. Repair of chronic distal biceps brachii tendon rupture using free autogenous semitendinosus tendon. Clin Orthop Relat Res 1996;(323):188–91.

45. Hallam P, Bain GI. Repair of chronic distal biceps tendon ruptures using autologous hamstring graft and the Endobutton. J Shoulder Elbow Surg 2004; 13(6):648–51.

46. Sotereanos DG, Pierce TD, Varitimidis SE. A simplified method for repair of distal biceps tendon ruptures. J Shoulder Elbow Surg 2000;9(3):227–33.

47. Rutland RT, Dunbar RP, Bowen JD. The biceps squeeze test for diagnosis of distal biceps tendon ruptures. Clin Orthop 2005;437:128–31.

48. O'Driscoll SW, Goncalves LB, Dietz P. The hook test for distal biceps tendon avulsion. Am J Sports Med 2007;35(11):1865–9.

49. Miller TT, Adler RS. Sonography of tears of the distal biceps tendon. AJR Am J Roentgenol 2000;175: 1081–6.

50. Fitzgerald SW, Curry DR, Erickson SJ, et al. Distal biceps tendon injury: MRI diagnosis. Radiology 1994;191:203–6.

51. Williams BD, Schweitzer ME, Weishaupt D, et al. Partial tears of the distal biceps tendon: MR

appearance and associated clinical findings. Skeletal Radiol 2001;30:560–4.

52. Giuffre' BM, Moss MJ. Optimal positioning for MRI of the distal biceps brachii tendon: flexed abducted supinated view. AJR Am J Roentgenol 2004;182:944–6.

53. Lee HG. Traumatic avulsion of tendon of insertion of biceps brachii. Am J Surg 1951;82(2):290–2.

54. Bernstein AD, Breslow MJ, Jazrawi LM. Distal biceps tendon ruptures: a historical perspective and current concepts. Am J Orthop 2001;30:193–200.

55. Baker BE, Bierwagen D. Rupture of the distal tendon of the biceps brachii. Operative versus nonoperative treatment. J Bone Joint Surg Am 1985;67(3):414–7.

56. Pearl ML, Bessos K, Wong K. Strength deficits related to distal biceps tendon rupture and repair. A case report. Am J Sports Med 1998;26(2):295–6.

57. Rantanen J, Orava S. Rupture of the distal biceps tendon. A report of 19 patients treated with anatomic reinsertion, and a meta-analysis of 147 cases found in the literature. Am J Sports Med 1999;27(2):128–32.

58. Chillemi C, Marinelli M, De Cupis V. Rupture of the distal biceps brachii tendon: conservative treatment versus anatomic reinsertion–clinical and radiological evaluation after 2 years. Arch Orthop Trauma Surg 2007;127(8):705–8.

59. Aldridge JW, Bruno RJ, Strauch RJ, et al. Management of acute and chronic biceps tendon rupture. Hand Clin 2000;16(3):497–503.

60. Rettig AC. Traumatic elbow injuries in the athlete. Orthop Clin North Am 2002;33(3):509–22.

61. Postacchini F, Puddu G. Subcutaneous rupture of the distal biceps brachii tendon: a report of seven cases. J Sports Med 1975;15:81–90.

62. Klonz A, Loitz D, Wohler P, et al. Rupture of the distal biceps brachii tendon: isokinetic power analysis and complications after anatomic reinsertion compared with fixation to the brachialis muscle. J Shoulder Elbow Surg 2003;12:607–11.

63. Boyd HB, Anderson LD. A method for reinsertion of the distal biceps brachii tendon. J Bone Joint Surg Am 1961;43:1041–3.

64. Failla JM, Amadio PC, Morrey BF, et al. Proximal radioulnar synostosis after repair of distal biceps brachii rupture by the two-incision technique: report of four cases. Clin Orthop 1990;253:133–6.

65. Wysocki RW, Cohen MS. Radioulnar heterotopic ossification after distal biceps tendon repair: results following surgical resection. J Hand Surg [Am] 2007;32(8):1230–6.

66. Sotereanos DG, Sarris I, Chou KH. Radioulnar synostosis after the 2-incision biceps repair: a standardized treatment protocol. J Shoulder Elbow Surg 2004;13(4):448–53.

67. Lintner S, Fischer T. Repair of the distal biceps tendon using suture anchors and an anterior approach. Clin Orthop Relat Res 1996;(322):116–9.

68. Bain GI, Prem H, Heptinstall·RJ, et al. Repair of distal biceps tendon rupture: a new technique using the Endobutton. J Shoulder Elbow Surg 2000;9(2):120–6.

69. Kobayashi K, Bruno RJ, Cassidy C. Single anterior incision suture anchor technique for distal biceps tendon ruptures. Orthopedics 2003;26(8):767–70.

70. Greenberg JA, Fernandez JJ, Wang T, et al. Endo-Button-assisted repair of distal biceps tendon ruptures. J Shoulder Elbow Surg 2003;12(5):484–90.

71. Khan W, Agarwal M, Funk L. Repair of distal biceps tendon rupture with the Biotenodesis screw. Arch Orthop Trauma Surg 2004;124(3):206–8.

72. John CK, Field LD, Weiss KS, et al. Single-incision repair of acute distal biceps ruptures by use of suture anchors. J Shoulder Elbow Surg 2007;16(1):78–83.

73. Khan AD, Penna S, Yin Q, et al. Repair of distal biceps tendon ruptures using suture anchors through a single anterior incision. Arthroscopy 2008;24(1):39–45.

74. Sanchez-Sotelo J, Morrey BF, Adams RA, et al. Reconstruction of chronic ruptures of the distal biceps tendon with use of an Achilles tendon allograft. J Bone Joint Surg Am 2002;84(6):999–1005.

75. Kaplan FT, Rokito AS, Birdzell MG, et al. Reconstruction of chronic distal biceps tendon rupture with use of fascia lata combined with a ligament augmentation device: a report of 3 cases. J Shoulder Elbow Surg 2002;11(6):633–6.

76. Bayat A, Neumann L, Wallace WA. Late repair of simultaneous bilateral distal biceps brachii tendon avulsion with fascia lata graft. Br J Sports Med 1999;33(4):281–3.

77. Levy HJ, Mashoof AA, Morgan D. Repair of chronic ruptures of the distal biceps tendon using flexor carpi radialis tendon graft. Am J Sports Med 2000;28(4):538–40.

78. Giombini A, Innocenzi L, Di Cesare A, et al. Partial rupture of the distal biceps brachii tendon in elite waterpolo goalkeeper: a case report of conservative treatment. J Sports Med Phys Fitness 2007;47(1):79–83.

79. Dürr HR, Stäbler A, Pfahler M, et al. Partial rupture of the distal biceps tendon. Clin Orthop Relat Res 2000;(374):195–200.

80. El-Hawary R, Macdermid JC, Faber KJ, et al. Distal biceps tendon repair: comparison of surgical techniques. J Hand Surg [Am] 2003;28(3):496–502.

81. Johnson TS, Johnson DC, Shindle MK, et al. One- versus 2-incision technique for distal biceps tendon repair. HSS J 2008;4(2):117–22.

82. Pereira DS, Kvitne RS, Liang M, et al. Surgical repair of distal biceps tendon ruptures: a biomechanical

comparison of 2 techniques. Am J Sports Med 2002;
30(3):432–6.

83. Lemos SE, Ebramzedeh E, Kvitne RS. A new technique: in vitro suture anchor fixation has superior yield
strength to bone tunnel fixation for distal biceps
tendon repair. Am J Sports Med 2004;32(2):406–10.

84. Idler CS, Montgomery WH 3rd, Lindsey DP, et al.
Distal biceps tendon repair: a biomechanical
comparison of intact tendon and 2 repair techniques. Am J Sports Med 2006;34(6):968–74.

85. Krushinski EM, Brown JA, Murthi AM. Distal biceps
tendon rupture: biomechanical analysis of repair

strength of the Bio-Tenodesis screw versus suture
anchors. J Shoulder Elbow Surg 2007;16(2):218–23.

86. Spang JT, Weinhold PS, Karas SG. A biomechanical
comparison of EndoButton versus suture anchor
repair of distal biceps tendon injuries. J Shoulder
Elbow Surg 2006;15(4):509–14.

87. Mazzocca AD, Burton KJ, Romeo AA, et al. Biomechanical evaluation of 4 techniques of distal biceps brachii tendon repair. Am J Sports Med 2007;35(2):252–8.

88. Blackmore SM, Jander RM, Culp RW. Management
of distal biceps and triceps ruptures. J Hand Ther
2006;19(2):154–68.

Arthroscopic Management of Scaphoid Fractures in Athletes

William B. Geissler, MD[a,b],*

KEYWORDS

- Scaphoid fracture • Scaphoid nonunion
- Arthroscopic fixation

The scaphoid is the most frequently fractured carpal bone in the wrist and accounts for approximately 70% of all carpal fractures.[1] This injury typically occurs in young adult men between the ages of 15 and 30 years.[2] In addition, the scaphoid fracture is a common athletic injury particularly in football and basketball, whereby aggressive play frequently causes impact injuries to the wrist. It is estimated that 1 out of 100 college football players will sustain a fracture of the scaphoid.[3] One common scenario involves an injured athlete who continues to compete and eventually presents to the treating physician with a scaphoid nonunion after the season is over.

Acute nondisplaced fractures of the scaphoid have traditionally been managed with cast and immobilization.[4,5] Nondisplaced scaphoid fractures have been reported to heal in 8 to 12 weeks when immobilized in long- and short-arm thumb spica casts.[4–6] The position of the wrist and whether a long- or short-arm thumb spica cast is the best treatment option is controversial if a scaphoid fracture is treated nonoperatively. The duration of cast and immobilization also varies dramatically according to the fracture site. A fracture of the scaphoid tubercle may be healed within a period of 6 weeks, whereas a fracture of the waist of the scaphoid may take three or more

months of immobilization. Fractures of the proximal third of the scaphoid may take 6 months or longer to heal with a cast due to the distal vascularity of the scaphoid.[7] Whereas nondisplaced fractures of the scaphoid are traditionally treated nonoperatively, the reported rate of nonunion for such fractures has been as high as 15%.[4–6]

Although cast and immobilization may be successful in up to 85% to 90% of cases, this may be at some cost to the patient, particularly an athlete, who may not be able to tolerate a lengthy course of immobilization during the season or while actively training. Prolonged immobilization may lead to muscle atrophy, disuse osteopenia, joint contracture, and financial hardship. An athlete may be inactive for 6 months or longer as the fracture unites.[6] This may result in a loss of a potential athletic scholarship or jeopardize his playing time on the team.

Displaced scaphoid fractures have a reported nonunion rate of up to 50%.[2] Fractures that decrease the prognosis for healing include the amount of displacement, the presence of associated carpal ligament instability, and delayed presentation greater than 4 to 6 weeks.[1] Acute displaced fractures of the scaphoid and scaphoid nonunions have traditionally been managed by open reduction and internal fixation.[1,2,8–16] This

[a] Section of Arthroscopic Surgery and Sports Medicine, Department of Orthopaedic Surgery and Rehabilitation, University of Mississippi Medical Center, 2500 North State Street, Jackson, MS 39216, USA
[b] Division of Hand and Upper Extremity Surgery, University of Mississippi Medical Center, Jackson, Mississippi
* Corresponding author. Section of Arthroscopic Surgery and Sports Medicine, Department of Orthopaedic Surgery and Rehabilitation, University of Mississippi Medical Center, 2500 North State Street, Jackson, MS 39216.
E-mail address: 3doghill@msn.com

Hand Clin 25 (2009) 359–369
doi:10.1016/j.hcl.2009.05.004
0749-0712/09/$ – see front matter © 2009 Published by Elsevier Inc.

requires significant soft tissue dissection. Complications have been reported, including avascular necrosis, carpal instability, donor site pain (bone graft), infection, screw protrusion, and reflex sympathetic dystrophy.[4,17] The most common reported complication in one series was hypertrophic scarring.[2] Jigs have been designed to assist in open reduction and in assisted arthroscopic reduction, but are difficult to apply, requiring further extensive surgical dissection.[18]

Wrist arthroscopy has revolutionized the practice of orthopedics by allowing the surgeon to examine and treat intra-articular abnormalities of the wrist joint under bright light and magnified conditions.[19] The scaphoid is well visualized from the radiocarpal and midcarpal spaces. Fractures of the scaphoid are best visualized with the arthroscope in the midcarpal space. Fractures of the waist of the scaphoid are best seen with the arthroscope in the radial midcarpal space, whereas fractures of the proximal pole are best visualized in the ulnar midcarpal space. Arthroscopic reduction of fractures of the scaphoid allows for direct visualization of the reduction of the scaphoid as the guide wires and percutaneous screws are being inserted. In addition, associated soft tissue injuries that may occur with a fracture of the scaphoid may be arthroscopically detected and managed at the same sitting.

This article reviews the indications and techniques for arthroscopic management of acute scaphoid fractures and nonunions. Arthroscopic techniques provide direct visualization of the fracture reduction and potentially result in greater range of motion due to percutaneous techniques, which limit scarring. In addition, percutaneous techniques allow the athlete to potentially return to competition more quickly compared with standard open techniques, particularly when an athlete is in training or during the season.

INDICATIONS

Arthroscopic fixation may be performed in acute nondisplaced fractures of the scaphoid and in acute displaced fractures of the scaphoid that are reducible.[20,21] For nondisplaced acute fractures, the risks and benefits of arthroscopic stabilization versus cast and immobilization must be discussed with the athlete so that an informed decision can be made by the athlete and associated family members. In acute reducible scaphoid fractures, the fracture may be reduced by manipulation of the wrist in a traction tower or by joysticks inserted into the proximal and distal poles, with the reduction viewed with the arthroscope in the midcarpal space.

Arthroscopic stabilization of selective scaphoid nonunions may also be performed. In 2005 Slade and Geissler[22] published their radiographic classification of scaphoid nonunions (**Table 1**). Type I fractures are the result of a delayed presentation (ie, 4–12 weeks from injury). A delayed presentation is well known to be a risk factor for nonunions of the scaphoid. In Type II injuries, a fibrous union is present. A minimal fracture line is seen on plain radiographs. The lunate is neutral and there is no humpback deformity. In Type III injuries, minimal sclerosis is seen at the fracture site. Sclerosis is less than 1 mm in length, the lunate is not rotated, and no humpback deformity is seen on imaging studies. In Type IV injuries, cystic formation has occurred. The area of cyst formation is between 1 and 5 mm. In Type IV injuries, a humpback deformity is not present and no rotation of the lunate is seen on plain radiographs. In Type V injuries, cystic changes are greater than 5 mm, and humpback deformity may be seen on plain radiographs or CT evaluation. The lunate has rotated into a dorsal intercalated segmental instability (DISI) position. In Type VI injuries, secondary degenerative changes are present with spurring along the radial border of the scaphoid and peaking of the radial styloid (scaphoid nonunion advanced collapse [SNAC]). Arthroscopic stabilization of scaphoid nonunions is indicated in Types I to IV. Once a humpback deformity is present, the arthroscopic stabilization is not recommended, and open reduction is suggested to correct the humpback deformity and rotation of the lunate.

PREOPERATIVE EVALUATION

Posterior-anterior and lateral radiographs are mandatory to assess displacement, alignment, and angulation of a fracture to the scaphoid. In addition, semi-pronated and supinated views are helpful to demonstrate the proximal and distal

Table 1 Scaphoid nonunion classification	
Slade and Geissler	
Type I	Delayed presentation 4–12 weeks
Type II	Fibrous union, minimal fracture line
Type III	Minimal sclerosis <1 mm
Type IV	Cystic formation, between 1 and 5 mm
Type V	Humpback deformity, >5 mm cystic change
Type VI	Wrist arthrosis

poles of the scaphoid, respectively. In posterior-anterior radiographs it is helpful to place the wrist in ulnar deviation, which extends the scaphoid for detection of fracture displacement. It is well recognized that a nondisplaced scaphoid fracture may not be present on initial radiographs for several weeks. It is important to immobilize the patient who presents with snuffbox tenderness until the pain resolves or until a diagnosis has been confirmed radiographically. In the athlete, for whom early diagnosis may be imperative during the season, MRI, or bone scan evaluation may be indicated when early detection of the scaphoid fracture is important.

CT parallel to the longitudinal axis of the scaphoid is used to evaluate displacement, angulation, and healing when further information is required to assess the fracture. In this technique, the patient is placed prone with the arms extended overhead and the wrist radial deviated to obtain the longitudinal axis of the scaphoid. Coronal slices are performed with supination of the forearm to a neutral position. CT evaluation is particularly important when nonoperative management of a scaphoid fracture is selected. It is difficult by plain radiography to judge healing of the scaphoid when treated nonoperatively. This evaluation is important, particularly in contact athletes, in making a decision when to return to play.

SURGICAL TECHNIQUES

Various arthroscopic-assisted and percutaneous techniques for fractures of the scaphoid have been previously described in the literature.[20–32] These include a volar approach popularized by Haddad and Goddard,[24] and the dorsal approach more recently popularized by Slade.[26] In general, these techniques include a small amount of wrist arthroscopy and a significant amount of fluoroscopy.

Volar Percutaneous Approach

The volar percutaneous approach was popularized by Haddad and Goddard.[24] Using this technique, the athlete is placed supine with arms suspended in a Chinese finger trap. Placing the thumb in suspension causes ulnar deviation of the wrist, which improves access to the distal pole of the scaphoid. Under fluoroscopic control, a longitudinal 0.5-cm incision is made on the most distal radial aspect of the scaphoid. Blunt dissection is used to expose the distal pole of the scaphoid. A percutaneous guide wire is introduced into the scaphoid trapezial joint and advanced proximally and dorsally across the fracture site. The position of the guide wire is checked

under fluoroscopy on anterior, posterior, oblique, and lateral planes. With the thumb in traction, the wrist can be rotated to provide nearly a 360° view of the position of the guide wire in the scaphoid. The length of the guide wire within the scaphoid is determined with a depth gauge, and a drill is inserted through a soft tissue protector to protect the surrounding tissues. One must bear in mind that the volar percutaneous approach is not benign. Blunt dissection and drilling of the scaphoid and insertion of screws should be used through a soft tissue protector to protect against injury to the surrounding cutaneous nerves and neurovascular structures. A headless cannulated screw is placed over the guide wire after drilling. A second guide wire is helpful to protect against rotation of fracture fragments while the screw is being inserted. Skin closure requires the use of a single suture, and the patient is encouraged to begin active finger flexion and extension exercises before discharge.

Haddad and Goddard[24] reported initial results in a pilot study of 15 patients with acute fractures of the scaphoid. Union was achieved in all patients within 57 days (range 38–71 days). The range of motion after union was equal to that of the contralateral limb and grip strength averaged 90% of the contralateral limb at 3 months with this percutaneous technique. The patients were able to return to sedentary work within 4 days and manual work within 5 weeks. The advantage of this technique is that it is fairly simple and requires minimal specialized equipment. With practice, the procedure can be done quickly. The potential disadvantage is that the screw is placed slightly obliquely to the mid waist fracture line in the scaphoid.

Dorsal Percutaneous Approach

Slade has popularized the dorsal percutaneous approach.[26,27] This technique has become popular because of its limited surgical dissection, and allows for arthroscopic evaluation and reduction of the fracture. The patient is placed supine on the table with the arm extended. Several towels are placed under the elbow to support the forearm so it is parallel to the floor. The wrist is flexed and pronated under fluoroscopy until the proximal distal poles of the scaphoid are aligned to form a perfect cylinder. Continuous fluoroscopy is recommended as the wrist is flexed to obtain a true ring sign as the proximal and distal poles align. Under fluoroscopy, a 14-gauge needle is placed percutaneously in the center of the ring sign and parallel to the beam of the fluoroscopy unit. The guide wire is then driven across the central axis of the scaphoid from dorsal to volar until the distal end of the guide wire comes in contact with the distal scaphoid cortex. The position of the guide wire is then evaluated under fluoroscopy in the posterior-anterior (PA), oblique, and lateral planes while maintaining the wrist in flexion. The wrist must not be extended as this could bend the guide wire. A second guide wire is then placed parallel to the first so it touches the tip of the proximal pole of the scaphoid cortex. The difference between the two lengths of the guide wires is the resulting length of the scaphoid.

Once the screw length has been determined, the primary guide wire is advanced volarly through a portion of the trapezium along the radial side of the thumb metacarpal to exit the skin on the volar aspect of the hand. The wire continues to be advanced out volarly until it is flush with the proximal pole of the scaphoid dorsally. Now the wrist can be extended without damage to the articular cartilage of the radiocarpal space.

The wrist is suspended in a traction tower, and the wrist can be evaluated from the radiocarpal and midcarpal space. Fracture reduction of the scaphoid is best judged with the arthroscope in the midcarpal space. Once the reduction is felt to be satisfactory as viewed arthroscopically, the primary guide wire is then advanced back proximally from volar to dorsal into the proximal pole of the scaphoid. The wrist is then flexed and the guide wire is advanced back out dorsally so that it protrudes from the skin. A portion of the wire is left out on the volar and dorsal aspects of the hand and wrist so that if the guide wire breaks, easy access to it is obtained. Blunt dissection is continued around the guide wire to ensure there is no soft tissue in a position of potential injury to the tendons as the scaphoid is drilled and the screw is inserted. Once the scaphoid has been reamed over the guide wire, a headless cannulated screw is then inserted over the guide wire to the depth previously reamed.

The dorsal approach has the advantage that the screw is able to be inserted down the central axis of the scaphoid. This action allows for compression directly across the fracture site compared with the more oblique potential insertion with the volar technique. The concern with the dorsal percutaneous approach is that the wrist is hyperflexed, and this may potentially displace the scaphoid fracture into a humpback deformity if it is unstable. It is important to evaluate the reduction of the scaphoid fracture with the arthroscope in the midcarpal portal when this technique is used, to ensure that the fracture is not hyperflexed.

Geissler and Slade[32] described using Slade's dorsal percutaneous fixation technique in 15 patients with stable fibrous nonunions of the scaphoid. In their series there were 12 horizontal oblique fractures, one transverse fracture, and two proximal pole fractures. The average presentation time to the clinic following injury was 8 months. All patients underwent percutaneous dorsal fixation with a headless cannulated screw and no accessory bone grafting procedure. In their series all 15 patients healed within 3 months on average. Eight of the 15 patients underwent CT evaluation to further document healing. The patients had an excellent range of motion at the final follow-up visit due to minimal surgical dissection. Using the modified Mayo wrist scale, 12 of 15 patients had excellent results. Dorsal percutaneous fixation was recommended for those patients with stable fibrous nonunions without any signs of humpback deformity and without extensive sclerosis of the fracture site. Using the scaphoid nonunion classification scale as proposed by Slade and Geissler, patients with Type II and Type III scaphoid nonunions were included in the study, with 100% success rate.

Arthroscopic Reduction (Geissler Technique)

Most recently Geissler[34] described his arthroscopic technique for reduction of acute scaphoid fractures in selective scaphoid nonunions (**Fig. 1**). The advantage of this technique is that the starting point for the guide wire is viewed directly arthroscopically. There is no guess work as to where the exact starting point for the guide wire or screw will be. In the author's opinion, this is a simpler approach than the dorsal

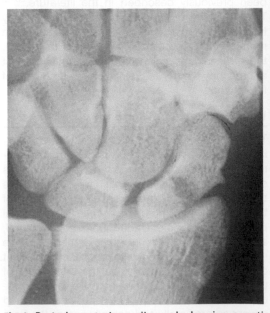

Fig. 1. Posterior-anterior radiograph showing a cystic scaphoid nonunion of the mid waist of the scaphoid.

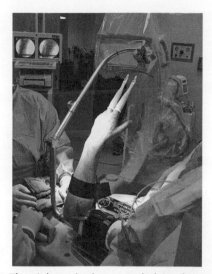

Fig. 2. The right wrist is suspended in the Acumed (Hillsboro, Oregon) wrist traction tower. The wrist is flexed approximately 30°.

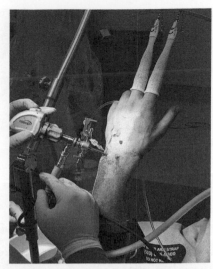

Fig. 4. The arthroscope is transferred into the 6-R portal, and the proximal pole of the scaphoid is visualized by looking across the wrist.

percutaneous approach with the ring sign. In addition, the wrist is not hyperflexed, which could potentially distract the scaphoid fracture fragments and cause a humpback deformity.

In this technique, the wrist is initially suspended in the wrist traction tower (Acumed, Hillsboro, OR, USA) (**Fig. 2**) The arthroscope is initially placed in the 3-4 portal to evaluate any associated soft tissue lesions which may occur with a scaphoid fracture (**Fig. 3**). On evaluation and treatment of

any associated soft tissue injuries, the arthroscope is then transferred into the 6-R portal. (**Fig. 4**) The wrist is flexed to approximately 30° in the traction tower. A 14-gauge needle is then inserted through the 3-4 portal, and the junction of the scapholunate interosseous ligament is palpated at its insertion onto the scaphoid (**Fig. 5**). The junction of the scapholunate interosseous ligament onto the scaphoid at its middle third is the most ideal point for screw entry. The 14-gauge needle is then

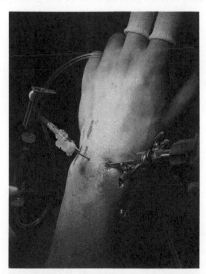

Fig. 3. The arthroscope is initially placed in the 3-4 portal to evaluate for any intercarpal soft tissue injuries associated with a scaphoid fracture. A needle is used to identify the precise location for the 6-R portal.

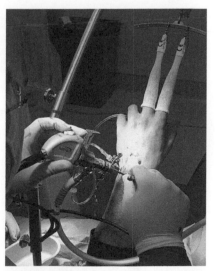

Fig. 5. A 14-gauge spinal needle is brought into the 3-4 portal. The junction of the scapholunate interosseous ligament to the proximal pole of the scaphoid is palpated.

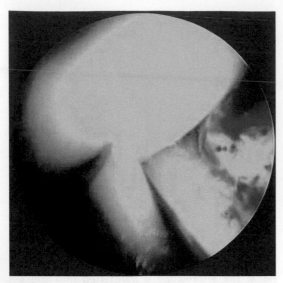

Fig. 6. The needle is impaled into the proximal pole of the scaphoid at the insertion of the scapholunate interosseous ligament.

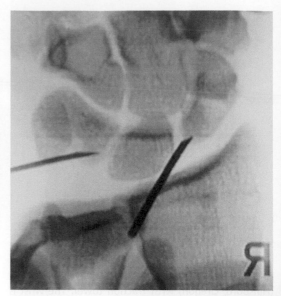

Fig. 8. Fluoroscopic view showing the ideal starting point on the proximal pole of the scaphoid.

advanced and impales into the most proximal aspect of the scaphoid right at the insertion of the scapholunate interosseous ligament (**Fig. 6**). Some dorsal synovium may occasionally block visualization of the starting point. It is important to debride the synovium so as to improve visualization.

The traction tower is flexed and the starting point of the needle is evaluated under fluoroscopy (**Fig. 7**). The starting point is consistently determined at the most proximal pole of the scaphoid

using this technique (**Fig. 8**). The needle is then simply aimed toward the thumb, and a guide wire is advanced through the needle down the central axis of the scaphoid to abut the distal pole (**Fig. 9**). The position of the guide wire is evaluated on the PA, oblique, and lateral planes under fluoroscopy (**Fig. 10**). This evaluation is done by rotating the forearm in the traction tower as the fluoroscopic image is not hindered by the support beam of the tower, which is to the side. A second guide wire is then placed against the proximal pole

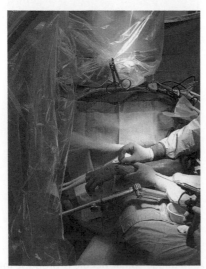

Fig. 7. The traction tower is flexed down to fluoroscopically confirm the starting point of the guide wire.

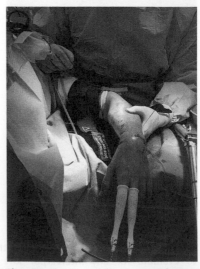

Fig. 9. The 14-gauge needle is aimed toward the thumb and a guide wire is placed down the central axis of the scaphoid.

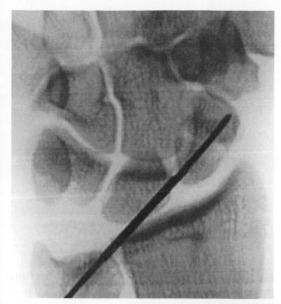

Fig.10. Fluoroscopic confirmation of the ideal position of the guide wire within the scaphoid on the poste-rior-anterior view.

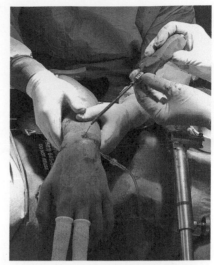

Fig. 11. The ideal length of the headless cannulated screw has been determined, and the guide wire has been advanced out of the volar aspect of the hand. The near cortex of the scaphoid is then reamed.

of the scaphoid. The difference in length is measured between the guide wires to obtain the length of the scaphoid screw. Just as in the dorsal percutaneous approach, a screw at least 4 mm shorter is recommended. Reduction of the scaphoid is evaluated with the arthroscope in the radial and possibly the ulnar midcarpal portals. If reduction is not satisfactory, the guide wire may continue to be advanced volarly across the fracture site, but still in the distal pole of the scaphoid. An additional Kirschner wire may then be placed on the dorsum of the proximal pole of the scaphoid. These wires can then be used as joysticks to further reduce the fracture anatomically as viewed directly with the arthroscope in the midcarpal portal. Also, manipulation of the tower, usually with the wrist in extension, further reduces the fracture. If the reduction is satisfactory, the guide wire is advanced out of the volar aspect of the wrist.

In acute scaphoid fractures or unstable fibrous nonunions, demineralized bone matrix putty is not used. A headless cannulated screw is inserted over the guide wire then across the fracture site. The position of the screw is checked in the PA, oblique, and lateral planes under fluoroscopy in the traction tower. The wrist is reevaluated arthroscopically from the radiocarpal and midcarpal spaces. From the radiocarpal space the surgeon must check that the headless screw is inserted up into the scaphoid and does not protrude to potentially injure the articular cartilage of the

scaphoid facet and the distal radius. The final reduction of the scaphoid fracture with the screw in place may be evaluated with the arthroscope in the midcarpal space.

In a scaphoid nonunion, percutaneous cancellous bone grafting or injection of demineralized bone matrix putty is performed. The scaphoid is reamed through a soft tissue protector (**Figs. 11** and **12**). A bone biopsy needle may then be filled with demineralized bone matrix or cancellous bone graft (**Fig. 13**). The bone biopsy needle is then placed over the guide wire from dorsal to proximal and inserted through the drill hole to the

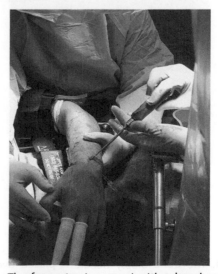

Fig. 12. The far cortex is reamed with a hand reamer.

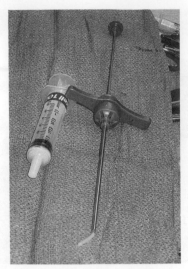

Fig.13. Accell putty (DBM, Irvine, California) is injected into a bone biopsy needle.

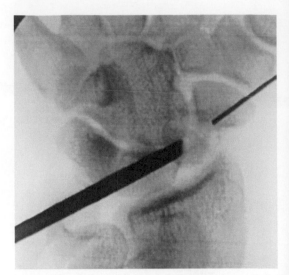

Fig. 15. The guide wire is advanced volarly, and the putty is injected directly into the cystic scaphoid nonunion site.

nonunion site (**Fig. 14**). The guide wire is retracted distally out of the proximal pole of the scaphoid remaining in the distal scaphoid (**Fig. 15**). The demineralized bone matrix is then injected by the bone biopsy needle into the central hole of the scaphoid at the nonunion site. With the bone biopsy needle still within the central canal of the scaphoid, the guide wire is advanced back from distal to proximal through the needle proximally and out of the dorsal skin. The bone biopsy needle is then removed (**Figs. 16** and **17**). In this manner, the guide wire has gone through the original path of the reamed scaphoid. A headless cannulated screw may then be inserted over the guide wire

across the scaphoid nonunion (**Figs. 18** and **19**). The radiocarpal and midcarpal spaces are now reevaluated arthroscopically to confirm the reduction and placement of the screw (**Fig. 20**).

Geissler recently described his technique of arthroscopic reduction of cystic scaphoid nonunions without humpback deformity, 34 with insertion of demineralized bone matrix (DBM) putty. Using the scaphoid nonunion classification scale of Slade and Geissler, his series comprised Type IV scaphoid nonunions. In his technique, 1 cm^3 of demineralized bone matrix (DBM-Accell,

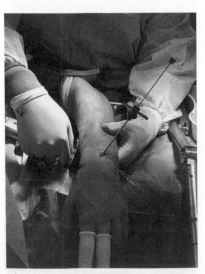

Fig. 14. The bone biopsy needle is placed over the guide wire at the level of the scaphoid nonunion.

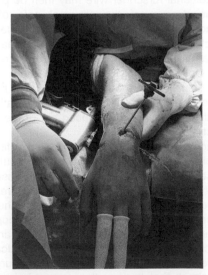

Fig. 16. Following injection of the putty, the guide wire is advanced back out dorsally through the cannula of the bone biopsy needle.

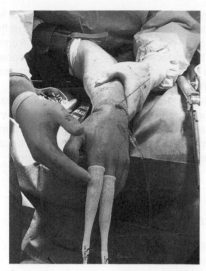

Fig. 17. The guide wire exits on the dorsal aspect of the wrist.

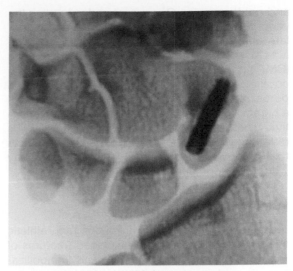

Fig. 19. Fluoroscopic confirmation of the placement of the headless cannulated screw across the fracture site.

Isotis, Irving, CA) was injected percutaneously in the nonunion site of the scaphoid. Fourteen of the 15 patients had their scaphoid nonunions healed using this technique. Arthroscopic evaluation of the wrist from the radiocarpal and midcarpal spaces showed no extravasation of the DBM putty into the joint.

Demineralized bone matrix is allograft bone that has been demineralized. The bone morphogenetic proteins (BMP) are preserved following the demineralization process. The entire cascade of bone morphogenetic protein evokes conversion of the mesenchymal cells to the preosteoblast and

eventually to the osteoblast, which is involved in bone formation. The advantage of demineralized bone matrix is that it involves the entire cascade of BMP rather than a single protein. When using small amounts of demineralized bone matrix one should note the carrier for the DBM and the percentage concentration of the DBM in the final product. Commercial providers may mix the DBM in carriers of different combinations and proportions. Products with a higher DBM content may be more effective because the active ingredient is the BMPs contained in the DBM itself

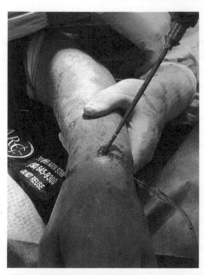

Fig. 18. The Acutrak II headless cannulated screw (Acumed, Hillsboro, Oregon) is inserted over the guide wire.

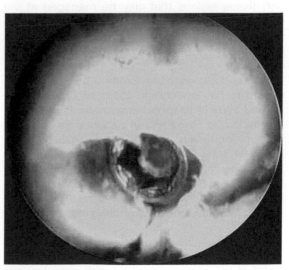

Fig. 20. Arthroscopic confirmation of the headless cannulated screw as inserted up into the scaphoid, and not prominent where it could potentially injure the articular cartilage of the scaphoid facet of the radius.

and not the carrier. One way of understanding the various BMP products is to imagine it as a chocolate chip cookie. The cookie itself is inert, which acts as a carrier for the sweet chocolate chips (BMPs). The more chocolate chips (BMP) in the cookie, the sweeter and better the cookie is perceived. Second-generation DBM putties have a higher content of BMPs and may be more effective. The surgeon should understand the various differences between the commercial products that are available so as to select a DBM putty with a high content of BMPs.

SUMMARY

Fractures of the scaphoid are a common athletic injury.[35] Whereas most nondisplaced fractures of the scaphoid will heal with cast and immobilization, nonunion rates of 10% to 15% have been reported.[4–6] This may severely affect an athlete's career if he has been immobilized for approximately 3 months, limiting his participation in athletics and training, and which still may result in a nonunion.

For this reason, arthroscopic fixation of acute scaphoid fractures in athletes is recommended once the advantages and disadvantages of the procedure have been discussed with the athlete and the family.[35,36] Cast and immobilization are effective but certainly may have disadvantages including muscle atrophy, joint contracture, and stiffness. Arthroscopic fixation of scaphoid fractures allows limited surgical dissection, which results in improved range of motion. Also, arthroscopic fixation allows for detection of associated soft tissue lesions that may be managed at the same sitting as the scaphoid fracture. Arthroscopic and percutaneous stabilization of acute scaphoid fractures has resulted in a high union rate.

Arthroscopic-assisted fixation has also been shown to be beneficial in cases of Type II, Type III, and Type IV scaphoid nonunions as described by Slade and Geissler.[22] In patients with a stable fibrous nonunion, potential stabilization with a screw alone has been shown to be effective.[33] In cystic changes, Geissler has shown good success with arthroscopic stabilization and percutaneous injection of DBM putty into the nonunion site.[34] Percutaneous bone grafting may be another option.

Arthroscopic fixation as described by Geissler limits the guesswork in locating the exact starting point of the screw compared with percutaneous fluoroscopic techniques.[37] The ideal starting point is at the most proximal pole of the scaphoid at the junction of the scapholunate interosseous ligament. It is reproducible, as confirmed fluoroscopically. In addition, the wrist is not hyperflexed, which may potentially flex the fracture fragments into a humpback deformity. The dorsal placement of the screw allows for central placement and compression of the fracture site.

Whether the scaphoid is reduced arthroscopically or percutaneously, these techniques are not indicated for those patients with severe humpback deformity with DISI rotation of the lunate or advanced arthrosis of the radiocarpal joint.

REFERENCES

1. Gelberman RH, Wolock BS, Siegel DB. Current concepts review: fractures and nonunions of the carpal scaphoid. J Bone Joint Surg Am 1989;71: 1560–5.
2. Cooney WP, Dobyns JH, Linscheid RL. Fractures of the scaphoid: a rational approach to management. Clin Orthop 1980;149:90–7.
3. Rettig AC, Ryan RO, Stone JA. Epidemiology of hand injuries in sports. In: Strickland JW, Rettig AC, editors. Hand injuries in athletes. Philadelphia: WB Saunders; 1992. p. 37–48.
4. Gellman H, Caputo RJ, Carter V, et al. Comparison of short and long thumb spica casts for nondisplaced fractures of the carpal scaphoid. J Bone Joint Surg Am 1989;71:354–7.
5. Kaneshiro SA, Failla JM, Tashman S. Scaphoid fracture displacement with forearm rotation in a short arm thumb spica cast. J Hand Surg 1989;71:354–7.
6. Skirven T, Trope J. Complications of immobilization. Hand Clin 1994;10:53–61.
7. Gelberman RH, Menon J. The vascularity of the scaphoid bone. J Hand Surg 1980;5:508–13.
8. Rettig AC, Weidenbener EJ, Gloyeske R. Alternative management of mid-third scaphoid fractures in the athlete. Am J Sports Med 1994;22:711–4.
9. DeMaagd RL, Engber WD. Retrograde Herbert screw fixation for treatment of proximal pole scaphoid nonunions. J Hand Surg 1989;14: 996–1003.
10. Filan SL, Herbert TJ. Herbert screw fixation of scaphoid fractures. J Bone Joint Surg 1996;78: 519–29.
11. Herbert TJ, Fisher WE. Management of the fractured scaphoid using a new bone screw. J Bone Joint Surg 1984;66:114–23.
12. O'Brien L, Herbert TJ. Internal fixation of acute scaphoid fractures: a new approach to treatment. Aust N Z J Surg 1985;55:387–9.
13. Rettig ME, Raskin KB. Retrograde compression screw fixation of acute proximal pole scaphoid fractures. J Hand Surg 1999;24:1206–10.

14. Russe O. Fracture of the carpal navicular: diagnosis, nonoperative treatment and operative treatment. J Bone Joint Surg 1960;42A:759.

15. Toby EB, Butler TE, McCormack TJ, et al. A comparison of fixation screws for the scaphoid during application of cyclic bending loads. J Bone Joint Surg 1997;79:1190–7.

16. Trumble TE, Clarke T, Kreder HJ. Nonunion of the scaphoid: treatment with cannulated screws compared with treatment with Herbert screws. J Bone Joint Surg 1996;78:1829–37.

17. Garcia-Elias M, Vall A, Salo JM, et al. Carpal alignment after different surgical approaches to the scaphoid: a comparative study. J Hand Surg 1988; 13:604–12.

18. Adams BD, Blair WF, Regan DS, et al. Technical factors related to Herbert screw fixation. J Bone Joint Surg 1988;13:893–9.

19. Whipple TL. The role of arthroscopy in the treatment of intraarticular wrist fractures. Hand Clin 1995;11:13–8.

20. Geissler WB. Arthroscopic assisted fixation of fractures of the scaphoid. Atlas Hand Clin 2003;8:37–56.

21. Geissler WB, Hammit MD. Arthroscopic aided fixation of scaphoid fractures. Hand Clin 2001;17:575–88.

22. Slade JF, Merrell GA, Geissler WB. Fixation of acute and selected nonunion scaphoid fractures. In: Geissler WB, editor. Wrist arthroscopy. New York: Springer; 2005. p. 112–24.

23. Cosio MQ, Camp RA. Percutaneous pinning of symptomatic scaphoid nonunions. J Hand Surg 1986;11:350–5.

24. Haddad FS, Goddard NJ. Acute percutaneous scaphoid fixation: a pilot study. J Bone Joint Surg 1998;80:95–9.

25. Shin A, Bond A, McBride M, et al. Acute screw fixation versus cast immobilization for stable scaphoid fractures: a prospective randomized study. Presented at American Society Surgery for the Hand, Seattle, October 5–7, 2000.

26. Slade JF III, Grauer JN, Mahoney JD. Arthroscopic reduction and percutaneous fixation of scaphoid fractures with a novel dorsal technique. Orthop Clin North Am 2000;30:247–61.

27. Slade JF III, Jaskwhich J. Percutaneous fixation of scaphoid fractures. Hand Clin 2001;17:553–74.

28. Taras JS, Sweet S, Shum W, et al. Percutaneous and arthroscopic screw fixation of scaphoid fractures in the athlete. Hand Clin 1999;15:467–73.

29. Slade JF III, Grauer JN. Dorsal percutaneous repair of scaphoid fractures with arthroscopic guidance. Atlas Hand Clin 2001;6:307–23.

30. Wozasek GE, Moser KD. Percutaneous screw fixation of fractures of the scaphoid. J Bone Joint Surg 1991;73:138–42.

31. Kamineni S, Lavy CBD. Percutaneous fixation of scaphoid fractures: an anatomic study. J Hand Surg 1999;24:85–8.

32. Geissler WB, Slade JF. Arthroscopic fixation of scaphoid nonunions without bone grafting. Presented American Society Surgery of the Hand, Phoenix, AZ, September 22, 2002.

33. Geissler WB. Arthroscopic fixation of cystic scaphoid nonunions with DBM. Presented American Association Hand Surgery, Tucson, AZ, January 17, 2006.

34. Geissler WB. Carpal fractures in athletes. Clin Sports Med 2001;20:167–88.

35. Rettig AC, Kollias SC. Internal fixation of acute stable scaphoid fractures in the athlete. Am J Sports Med 1996;24:182–6.

36. Geissler WB. Wrist arthroscopy. New York: Springer; 2005.

37. Fernandez DL. Anterior bone grafting and conventional lag screw fixation to treat scaphoid nonunions. J Hand Surg Am 1990;15:140–7.

Carpal Fractures in Athletes Excluding the Scaphoid

Jeffrey Marchessault, MD*, Matt Conti, BS, Mark E. Baratz, MD

KEYWORDS

- Triquetrum • Trapezoid • Trapezium
- Lunate • Capitate • Pisiform • Hamate

A wide range of hand and wrist injuries occur in today's recreational and elite athletes and account for 3% to 9% of all sports injuries.[1–4] The onus is on the physician to discriminate between injuries that can be managed with an early return to sport and those injuries that place the athlete at risk of further injury if not managed aggressively from the outset. The physician and the athlete must understand the balance between safe, early return to sport, and prompt surgical treatment that prevents late disability.

TRIQUETRAL FRACTURES
Incidence

Triquetral fractures are second only to scaphoid fractures as the most common carpal fractures, comprising 3% to 5% of all carpal fractures.[5–8] Two primary fracture patterns are observed; a dorsal chip or cortical fracture and triquetral body fractures. The dorsal chip fracture is much more common, reported to be as high as 93% of all triquetral fractures.[7] Triquetral body fractures more commonly infer a high amount of energy to the wrist, and are observed with perilunate fracture dislocations in 12% to 25% of triquetrum injuries.[6,9–11]

Mechanism of Injury

Different mechanisms have been proposed for dorsal triquetrum fractures. Extreme palmar flexion with radial deviation is believed to cause the dorsal avulsion fracture at the attachment of the strong radiotriquetral and triquetroscaphoid ligaments.[8,12] The more common clinical presentation is a fall onto an ulnarly deviated wrist in dorsiflexion. Wrist dorsiflexion and ulnar deviation has been shown to drive the ulnar styloid as a chisel into the dorsal cortex of the triquetrum.[13–15] Large styloid size has been proposed as a predisposition to this fracture pattern.[15] The chisel action of the proximal edge of the hamate against the distal triquetrum during wrist extension has also been proposed to explain these dorsal triquetrum chip fractures.[7]

Triquetrum body fractures often involve high-energy injuries to the hand and are associated with greater arc perilunate fracture dislocations.[16] Triquetrum fractures alone, with a history of violent collision, should alert the physician to seek out potential ligament injuries around the carpus as 12% to 25% of triquetrum fractures are associated with perilunate fracture dislocations.[17] The more obvious scaphoid fracture seen in the transscaphoid perilunate fracture dislocation, the most common greater arc pattern, can draw attention away from a concomitant triquetrum fracture (**Fig. 1**).[18] Triquetral fractures can also be seen concurrently with fractures of the hamate, distal ulna, or distal radius.[5,7]

Examination

Point tenderness solely over the triquetrum is difficult to elicit in the acute setting given the proximity of the triangular fibrocartilage complex (TFCC) and other ulnar wrist structures. Pain with wrist flexion

Department of Orthopaedic Surgery, Allegheny General Hospital, 1307 Federal Street, 2nd Floor, Pittsburgh, PA 15212, USA

* Corresponding author.
E-mail address: jeffrey-marchess@hotmail.com (J. Marchessault).

Hand Clin 25 (2009) 371–388
doi:10.1016/j.hcl.2009.05.013
0749-0712/09/$ – see front matter © 2009 Elsevier Inc. All rights reserved.

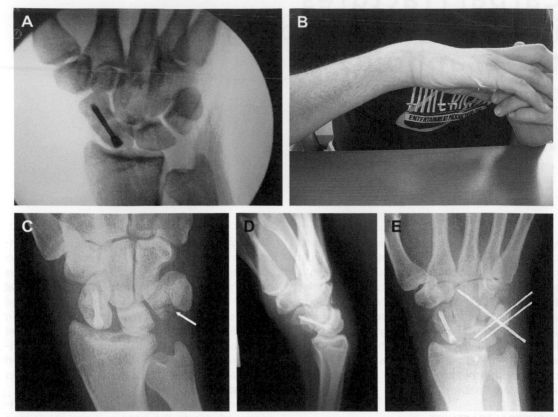

Fig. 1. (*A–E*) A 22-year-old man suffered transscaphoid perilunate fracture dislocation of the wrist. The wrist was reduced in the emergency department and was well aligned with the exception of the scaphoid. The scaphoid was fixed and again the carpus was well aligned on the PA view (*A*) and lateral view. No further treatment was given. At the first postoperative visit he complained of wrist pain and deformity. The wrist was held in a position of flexion (*B*). The PA radiograph shows a triangular appearing lunate and displaced fracture of the trique-trum (*arrow*) (*C*). The lateral radiograph shows a marked VISI deformity resulting from the untreated triquetral fracture with associated lunotriquetral instability (*D*). The PA radiographs after open reduction and pinning of the lunotriquetral ligament and midcarpal joint along with indirect reduction of the triquetral fracture on the radial palmer aspect of the triquetrum (*E*).

and extension is present with dorsal avulsion injuries.

Radiographic Evaluation

Many triquetral fractures can be identified with an-teroposterior, lateral and 45-degree pronated obli-que radiographs of the wrist.[11,13] The lateral and oblique views often reveal the dorsal cortical frac-tures. CT scans are helpful in identifying occult tri-quetral fractures.

Treatment

A dorsal chip fracture is a common incidental finding on the lateral radiograph of an injured athlete. It is useful to determine if the fracture is acute or chronic, and if the recent injury has a mechanism consistent with a triquetral fracture. If all evidence points to an acute injury, the athlete

needs to understand that the fracture itself has little consequence. It is the underlying soft-tissue injury that must be treated because the fracture will, most likely, go on to an asymptomatic, fibrous union. Various investigators have recommended immobilization, usually with a short arm cast, for 3 to 6 weeks.[5,7,19,20] The authors try to tailor the treatment to the athlete and the injury. If the wrist is markedly swollen, there is a significant soft-tissue injury that will preclude a rapid return to sports. The wrist is placed in a splint and an MR is obtained to identify extrinsic or intercarpal liga-ment injuries or occult fractures. In the absence of an obvious operable lesion, the wrist is re-examined in 1 week and usually protected with a cast. If there is negligible swelling and minimal tenderness at the first examination, athletes who do not require wrist motion for their sport are permitted to try to play with a wrist support. This approach must include frequent re-examination to ensure that play is not exacerbating the underlying injury. For injuries in between, short periods of immobilization (1–2 weeks) are preferred with re-examination to facilitate a safe early return to sport. When pain and stiffness persist beyond 8 weeks, MR arthrography is recommended to investigate the possibility of a concurrent intercarpal ligament injury or tear of the TFCC. Dorsal fractures that remain symptomatic can be treated by excision of the ununited fragment.[20] Symptoms emanating from the fragment alone are unusual.

Guidelines for treatment of triquetrum body fractures are less clear. In the setting of a concomitant wrist fracture dislocation, it is common to treat the lunotriquetral ligament injury by pinning the joint and ignoring the fracture to the triquetrum. In the rare instance of a displaced triquetral body fracture, open reduction and internal fixation has been described.[18,21] Pisiform excision has provided pain relief in patients presenting remote from their injury with a malunion, nonunion or post-traumatic pisotriquetral arthritis following a triquetrum body fracture.[22,23]

Complications

The most common complication of a triquetrum fracture is a misdiagnosis or delay in diagnosis. This complication can be avoided with a serial clinical and radiographic examination for athletes presenting with prolonged ulnar-sided wrist pain or tenderness over the triquetrum.

HAMATE FRACTURES
Incidence

Hamate fractures constitute approximately 2% of all carpal fractures.[24] The unique anatomy of the hamate hook places the bone at risk from compressive forces when the palm is struck and shear forces from the adjacent flexor tendons arise during forceful torque of the wrist.[25] The hamate forms the radial border of Guyon's canal and the ulnar border of the carpal tunnel (**Fig. 2**). Injury to the hamate can result in median and ulnar nerve dysfunction, although symptoms of median nerve dysfunction are rare. The diagnosis of hamate fractures can be clinically challenging with many fractures diagnosed long after injury.[26,27]

Mechanism of Injury

Hamate hook fractures occur from direct compressive forces, shear forces, or a combination of both. Both of these forces arise in tennis, in the baseball player when batting and in the golfer during a shot that is hit "fat." The nondominant hand is usually at risk in the batter or golfer. Dominant hands are

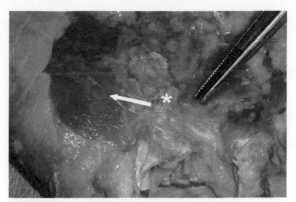

Fig. 2. The TCL forms the roof of the carpal canal (*forceps*) and the floor of Guyon's canal. Pull from the thenar muscles (*arrow*) through the TCL can displace a fractured hamate (*asterix*).

involved in tennis and other racquet sports when only one hand receives the force of impact. The taut flexor tendons at the base of the hamate exert shear forces during power grip in an ulnarly deviated wrist, as is seen in racquet sports.[24]

Hamate body fractures generally occur with a high-energy axial load to the fourth and fifth metacarpals resulting in a carpometacarpal (CMC) fracture dislocation.[19,28] Hamate body fractures have been classified as coronal or transverse.[29] Coronal plane fractures result from axial loads applied as described earlier.[30]

Examination

Pain in the ulnar palm aggravated by active grasp is the most common sign of a hamate hook fracture.[31] Tenderness to palpation is elicited directly over the hamate hook, 2 cm distal to the pisiform in line between the second metacarpal head and pisiform.[32] Occasionally, ulnar nerve paresthesias will be acutely present.[31] In delayed presentation, patients present with vague ulnar-sided wrist and hand pain,[31] median[33] or ulnar nerve[34] symptoms, and weakness of grip from affected ulnar-sided flexor tendons.[35] Pain with resisted ring and small finger flexion worsened with wrist ulnar deviation and lessened by radial deviation can uncover the occult hamate hook injury irritating the flexor tendons to the ring and small fingers (**Fig. 3**).[25] Flexor tendonitis of the ring or small fingers is uncommon in athletes. The possibility of a hamate hook fracture should be considered even in the absence of tenderness over the hook or in the face of normal wrist imaging. An unrecognized and untreated hamate hook fracture may lead to a partial or complete rupture of the IVth or Vth deep or superficial flexors (**Fig. 4**).

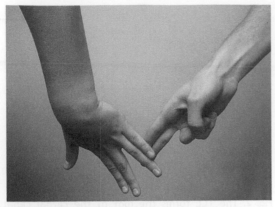

Fig. 3. The combination of wrist ulnar deviation and resisted wrist flexion can elicit pain from tendonitis emanating from a hook of the hamate fracture.

Imaging

Radiographic findings of hamate fractures on standard views of the hand are subtle. The PA radiograph of an uninjured wrist has an oblique articular space separating the distal margin of the hamate from the base of the IVth and Vth metacarpals (**Fig. 5**). This space is lost following a IVth or Vth CMC dislocation with a shear fracture of the anterior aspect of the hamate (**Fig. 6**).

The normal PA radiograph of the wrist also has a circular density at the distal margin of the hamate (**Fig. 7**). **Fig. 7** shows an end-on view of the hamate hook. Loss of this circle occurs with a displaced hamate hook fracture. Increased sclerosis about the circle can occur with a nondisplaced nonunion of the hamate hook.[36] Three specialized views; carpal tunnel view,[37] a supinated oblique view with the wrist dorsiflexed,[38,39] and a lateral view projected through the first web space with the

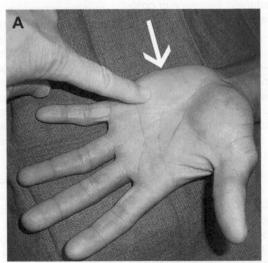

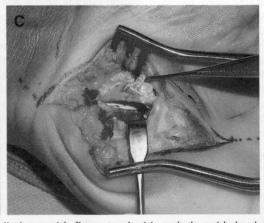

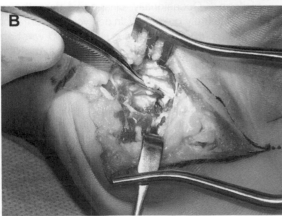

Fig. 4. Callous over the hypothenar eminence in a baseball player with flexor tendonitis and ulnar-sided palm pain (A). Fracture distal margin of the hamate at the CMC joint. The hamate hook was not fractured (B). Partial flexion tendon laceration from abrasion against the fractured hamate (C).

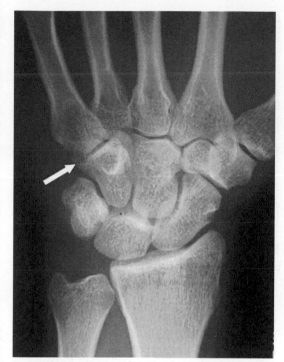

Fig. 5. Posteroanterior view of the wrist with a joint space clearly visible between the base of the fifth metacarpal and the hamate (*arrow*) and all of the other CMC joints.

thumb abducted,[40] have been described to bring the hamate hook into better view. The carpal tunnel view is commonly used for its reproducible profile of the hook (**Fig. 8**), but can be difficult to

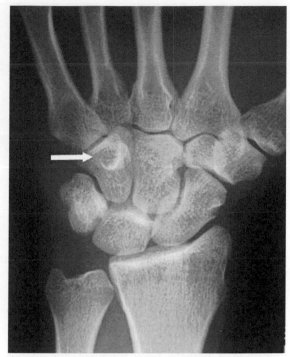

Fig. 7. Sclerotic circle on the PA view of the wrist results from an end-on view of the normal hamate hook (*arrow*).

obtain if fracture pain precludes sufficient wrist extension.

Studies have shown the superiority of CT imaging with the hands in the praying position for detecting occult hamate fractures.[41,42] The additional bone detail from a CT scan can also exclude congenital variations such as os hamuli proprium (**Fig. 9**).[18]

Treatment

Displaced fractures of the hamate body are best treated with operative reduction and internal fixation, particularly in the setting of a shear fracture occurring with a IVth or Vth CMC dislocation. The fracture is easily exposed between the IVth and Vth extensor digitorum communis tendons. Fixation of the fracture is best achieved with mini fragment screws. Care must be taken when drilling dorsal to the palmar through the hamate because the motor branch of the ulnar nerve hugs the ulnar and distal margins of the hamate hook (**Fig. 10**).[43]

Treatment options for acute hamate hook fractures include immobilization, open reduction, and internal fixation and excision. Although there is support in the literature for each option, in practice most fractures are treated with excision.

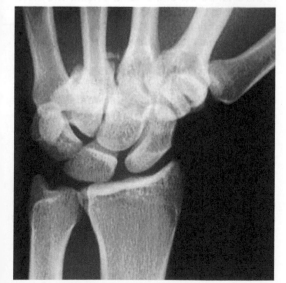

Fig. 6. Obliteration of CMC joint space in a patient with a III to V CMC fracture dislocation.

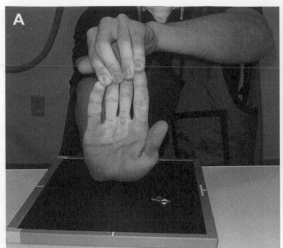
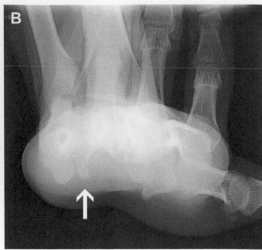

Fig. 8. Hand held in maximum extension to facilitate the carpal tunnel view (*A*). Carpal tunnel view with *arrow* showing the hamate hook (*B*).

Nonoperative management has been successful for nondisplaced hook fractures when diagnosed within the first week of injury.[44] Results are less favorable if hamate hook fractures are treated beyond the first week.[45] It has been suggested that slight wrist flexion with the IVth and Vth metacarpophalangeal joints in maximum flexion lessens the shear forces on the hook from the ulnar flexor tendons. Immobilizing the thumb is believed to minimize the pull of thenar muscles on the hook by the transverse carpal ligament (TCL) (**Fig. 2**).[46]

Proponents of open fixation of hamate hook fractures cite a cadaver study demonstrating loss of strength with removal of the hamate.[47] Although patients should be counseled on this possibility, weakness has not been a significant deficit in clinical studies.[48] Published literature on the results of

open reduction and internal fixation (ORIF) is scant. One review reported nonunion or questionable union in 4 out of 9 patients.[26]

Excision of acute hamate hook fractures is considered the optimal treatment of athletes attempting the earliest return to sport (**Fig. 11A**).[39] Exposure is accomplished through a curvilinear incision center over the hamate hook. Crossing the wrist crease should be avoided if possible. Anecdotal experience has suggested that scars in the wrist crease seem to remain sensitive longer than those in the palm. The ulnar nerve and artery are identified radial to the pisiform at the entrance to Guyon's canal. The nerve and artery are traced to the ulnar border of the hamate hook. The motor branch exits the ulnar nerve proper on the dorsal-ulnar aspect of the nerve and then passes dorsal to the ulnar nerve beneath the flexor digiti minimi[49] and around the distal ulnar border of the hamate hook. The motor branch must be mobilized and retracted before exposure of the hamate hook (see **Fig. 10**). The tip of the hook is palpated and is then exposed by elevating the periosteum. The hook is surprisingly long (**Fig. 11B**). Patience is required to safely expose the hook down to its base. Most fractures pass through the base of the hook. In all cases, even those with a fracture that is more anterior through the hook, removal of all of the hook is preferred. This procedure should prevent the remaining bone from irritating the flexor tendons.

A lateral approach has also been described for hamate hook excision. The incision is placed adjacent to the fifth metacarpal. The abductor and opponens digiti minimi are elevated to expose the base of the hamate hook.[50]

Fig. 9. CT view of the carpal canal illustrating a hamate hook fracture (*arrow*).

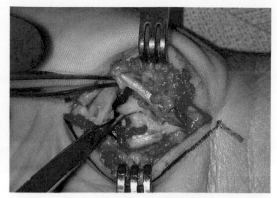

Fig. 10. Deep motor branch of the ulnar nerve (*tip of scissors*) as it passes around the base of the hook of the hamate.

Hamate hook excision is also the recommended treatment of symptomatic nonunions. Case series have demonstrated a predictable return to high levels of sports following excision of the hamate hook.[39,51]

Return to sports following hamate hook excision is generally quick, with scar sensitivity being the limiting factor. Gentle use of the hand is started immediately focusing on the finger range of motion. Sutures are removed at 10 to 14 days as the wound is managed with scar massage and a silicone patch. Light workouts including grip strengthening are permitted with a padded glove, such as a biking glove. Baseball players begin dry swings (no contact) with a bat. Golfers and racquet players can similarly practice swings without contact. Golfers can practice putting and chipping off a mat. At week three, baseball players begin hitting off a tee and progress to hitting pitches, as tolerated. Racquet players start light volleying and progress to ground strokes, as tolerated. Golfers progress from quarter to full swings hitting balls

off a mat during week three. In week four they progress from quarter to full swings hitting balls off the grass. Most athletes can return to their sport in 4 to 6 weeks. The scar sensitivity decreases over time, but does not go away for 4 to 6 months.

Complications

Rupture or fraying of the flexor digitorum profundus and superficialis tendons to the ring and small fingers at the irregular surface of the hamate fracture has been reported in a literature review of approximately 14% of cases.[26] Ruptured flexor tendons are repaired with palmaris tendon bridge grafts or end-to-side repairs.[26]

A water shed area of vascularization has been proposed to put the hamate hook fractures at risk for nonunion[52,53] as osteonecrosis of a hamate body[54] and hook[55] after fracture has been reported.

A 3% complication rate has been reported in association with excision of the hamate hook fractures[56] with nerve injury being the most common untoward event.

TRAPEZIUM FRACTURES
Incidence

Trapezium fractures comprise 4% to 5% of carpal fractures.[57–59] Fractures of the trapezium body are most common and described as horizontal and sagittal split, transarticular, dorsoradial tuberosity, and comminuted.[60] Sagittal split fractures are the most common. Volar trapezial ridge fractures, attachment site for the TCL, are less common. Ridge fractures have been classified as type I base fractures and type II avulsion tip fractures.[59] The association of trapezium fractures and first metacarpal fractures is well documented.[58,61,62] Other concomitant injuries include fractures of the scaphoid, distal radius, and hamate.[58,61,62]

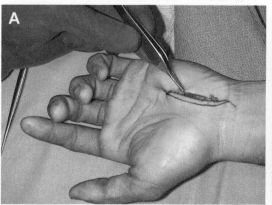
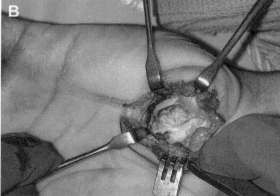

Fig. 11. Exposure of the hamate hook with a curvilinear incision in the palm centered over the hook of the hamate (*A*). Exposed hook of hamate (*B*).

Mechanism of Injury

The protected position of the trapezium below the first metacarpal often prevents direct blows from causing fractures. Many trapezium fractures are the result of high-energy injuries, particularly motor vehicle accidents.[61] These fractures also occur from a fall onto an outstretched hand whereby an axial load on the dorsiflexed wrist drives the metacarpal into the trapezium.[20] The radial styloid can also be driven into the trapezium if the wrist is radially deviated and the thumb is abducted and hyperextended. Lateral body fragments commonly remain attached to the first metacarpal by connecting ligaments, and displace radially and proximally from the pull of the abductor pollicis longus.[17]

Examination

Point tenderness at the volar base of the thumb, just distal to the volar tubercle of the scaphoid is a reliable finding in the acute setting. Painful and weakened pinch is also a telling sign. Pain is often exacerbated with wrist flexion due to the close proximity of the flexor carpi radialis (FCR) to the longitudinal groove adjacent to the volar ridge (**Fig. 12**).

Radiographic Evaluation

Standard views of the hand frequently reveal trapezium body fractures (**Fig. 13**). Bett's view, a pronated anterior-posterior view has been described to better visualize the trapeziometacarpal articulation.[17] The carpal canal view best demonstrates trapezial ridge fractures (**Fig. 14**).[63] CT is useful in chronic cases involving trauma to the wrist and for identifying occult ridge fractures or the rare coronal fracture (**Fig. 15**).[64]

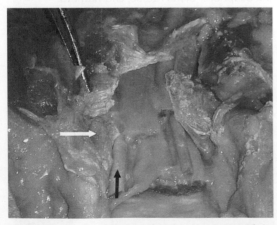

Fig. 12. Anatomic dissection showing proximity of the trapezial ridge (*white arrow*) to the FCR tendon (*black arrow*).

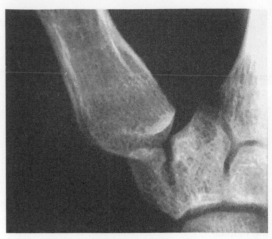

Fig. 13. Oblique view (pronated) view of the wrist reveals a longitudinal fracture of the body of the trapezium. (*Courtesy of* Michael Hayton, MD, Manchester, UK.)

Treatment

Nondisplaced trapezial body fractures can be treated with thumb spica immobilization for 4 to 6 weeks. Intraarticular fractures displaced 2 mm or more, are best exposed through a Wagner approach. An incision is made along the radial and proximal margins of the thenar musculature at the junction of the glaborous skin of the palm and the dorsal skin of the wrist (**Fig. 16**). The thenar muscles are elevated exposing the trapezium and thumb CMC joint. Care should be taken to protect the superficial radial nerve and radial artery.[65] Fixation is achieved with pin or mini fragment screws.[61] The goal of fixation is to minimize the risk of deformity and posttraumatic arthritis. A dynamic traction splint using oblique traction with a percutaneous wire through the first metacarpal attached to an outrigger has been devised in an attempt to permit early motion.[66]

Type I ridge fractures at the base can be treated nonoperatively with cast immobilization for 6 weeks. However, the pull of the TCL and the adjacent FCR may induce fracture motion that prevents healing.[67] Fracture excision has been recommended for type II ridge fractures given the high rate of nonunion (see **Fig. 14**).[59]

Complications

Patients with a missed trapezial fracture may develop irritation of the median nerve[67] or FCR tendon. Posttraumatic arthritis is a common radiographic finding after trapezial body fractures, but is frequently asymptomatic.[61]

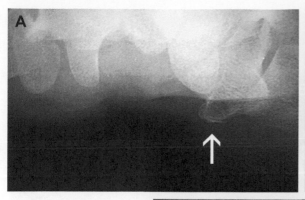
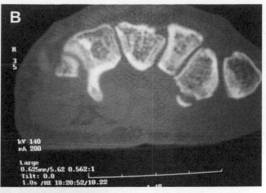
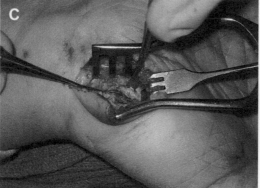

Fig. 14. (*A*) Carpal tunnel view demonstrating a fracture of the trapezial ridge (*arrow*). (*B*) CT scan demonstrating fracture of the trapezial ridge. (*C*) Incision near the base of the thenar eminence with resection of the fractured trapezial ridge.

CAPITATE FRACTURES
Incidence

Capitate fractures comprise 1% to 2% of all carpal fractures.[24] The capitate is protected in the center of the hand by the surrounding carpus bones and metacarpals. A high-energy injury is typically necessary to create a fracture. In one study, capitate fractures occurred four times more commonly as part of a perilunate fracture dislocation than in isolation.[68] The combination of scaphoid waist fracture and capitate fracture with malrotation of the proximal fragment has been called the naviculo-capitate or scaphocapitate, fracture syndrome.[69] The most common fracture pattern is the transscaphoid, transcapitate perilunate fracture dislocation.[68]

Mechanism of Injury

Isolated capitate fractures are believed to result from a direct blow or by an indirect axial load through the third metacarpal with the wrist flexed.[70] The latter mechanism results in a fracture at the neck of the capitate and base of the third metacarpal.[70]

A transscaphoid, transcapitate perilunate fracture dislocation is believed to occur with wrist hyperextension and radial deviation with the radial styloid striking the scaphoid.[69] Another proposed mechanism suggests that the dorsal lip of the distal radius strikes the dorsal surface of the capitate, flipping the unattached proximal pole fragment 180 degrees.[71,72]

Examination

Early diagnosis is aided with a high index of suspicion and careful palpation to localize tenderness dorsal to the fractured capitate.

Radiographic Evaluation

Standard anteroposterior, lateral, and oblique views of the hand often elucidate capitate fractures. Fractures in the coronal plane are better visualized by CT scan[73] or MRI.[74] Imaging with MRI may help assess surrounding ligaments. In practice, MRI is infrequently used in this setting because most of these injuries require surgical treatment by a dorsal approach allowing the surgeon to inspect the intercarpal and extrinsic ligaments, as well as the TFCC.

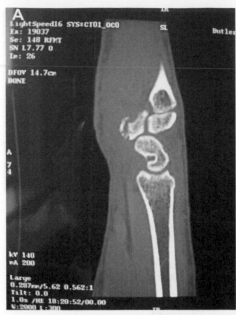
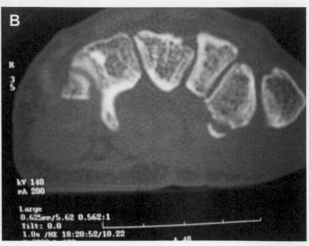

Fig. 15. CT revealing a coronal fracture through the body of the trapezium on sagittal (*A*) and axial (*B*) views.

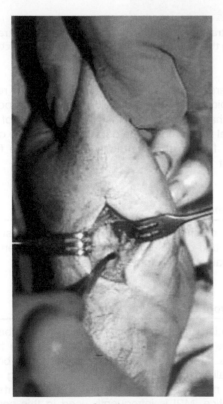

Fig. 16. Skin incision for the Wagner approach to trapezium body fractures is along the glaborous skin of the palm and the dorsal skin of the wrist. This approach places the branches of the radial artery and nerve at risk.

Treatment

Nonoperative treatment should only be pursued in nondisplaced neck fractures.

Discontinuation of the cast or splint is advised only after radiographic and clinical signs of healing are present. In those instances whereby plain radiographs provide equivocal evidence of healing, CT images in the coronal plain can be relied on to identify crossing trabecula.

ORIF with pins or compression screws is performed through a dorsal incision between the third and fourth extensor compartments in line with the radial border of the long finger.[20] Palmar flexion of the wrist improves access to the proximal fragment. Concomitant scaphoid fractures and scapholunate ligament repairs can be addressed through the same dorsal approach. Cannulated headless screws from proximal to distal in the capitate provide adequate stability to allow a range of motion in 2 weeks (**Fig. 17**).[20,75]

This injury has a varied prognosis that depends on the extent of injury to the soft tissues and to the articular surface, whether or not the head fragment heals or develops avascular necrosis (AVN). Midcarpal arthritis is a common consequence. Depending on the athlete's sport and response to treatment, this is typically a season-ending, if not a career-ending injury.

Complications

Early diagnosis is the key to success in properly treating capitate fractures. The retrograde

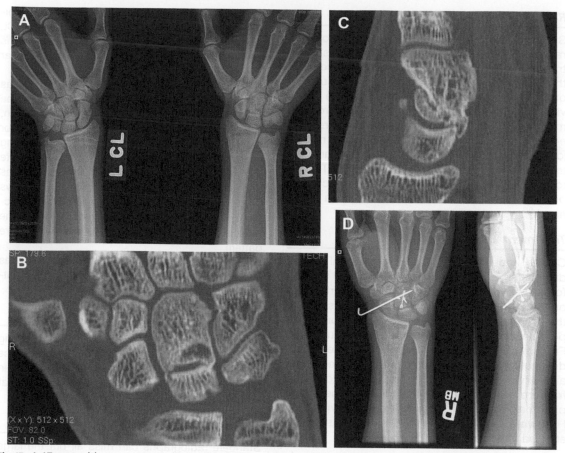

Fig. 17. A 17-year-old man presented 7 weeks after punching a tree, sustaining an isolated right capitate fracture seen on the plain radiographs (*A*), coronal and sagittal CT images (*B, C*). Postoperative radiograph of open reduction internal fixation with a headless compression screw (*D*). (*Courtesy of* Andrew W. Cross, MD, Cincinnati, OH.)

interosseous blood flow of the capitate is much like the scaphoid and places the proximal pole prone to AVN with fractures at mid-level.[76,77] Despite this tenuous blood supply, AVN of the proximal fragment has been reported infrequently in isolated capitate fractures if not associated with high-energy fracture dislocations.[77–80] Higher energy fracture dislocations place the proximal capitate at risk, especially when malrotated.[68,81] Nonunion of isolated capitate fractures occurs in more than 50% of cases.[17] AVN and painful nonunions can be addressed by corticocanellous bone grafts to restore carpal height and promote healing.[82]

As mentioned earlier, stiffness and midcarpal arthritis are common with intraarticular fractures of the wrist, particularly if the fracture occurs with a carpal dislocation.

TRAPEZOID FRACTURES
Incidence

Trapezoid fractures constitute less than 1% of carpal fractures.[26] Like the capitate, the trapezoid is protected by the surrounding metacarpal and carpal bones. Fractures of the trapezoid typically result from high-energy injuries to the hand. There are no series to guide treatment.

Mechanism of Injury

The trapezoid is keystone-shaped and the dorsal surface is twice that of the volar side. This shape, coupled with stronger volar than dorsal ligaments, predisposes the trapezoid to dorsal dislocation.[83] An axial force through the flexed second metacarpal exerts a palmarly directed force on the trapezoid, displacing it dorsally.[84] However, volar dislocation of the trapezoid has been described as a result of a high-energy injury to the hand.[85]

Examination

Point tenderness at the base of the index metacarpal, pain with motion and deformity can lead to the diagnosis. Pain can be elicited with gentle motion of the second metacarpal.

Radiographic Evaluation

Standard anteroposterior, lateral, and oblique radiographs often permit detection of isolated trapezoid dislocations. Fracture dislocations of the trapeziometacarpal joint are best visualized on the anteroposterior view rather than the lateral view. The dislocated trapezoid allows proximal migration of the second metacarpal. The proximal edge of the metacarpal will obscure the normal joint space between the distal scaphoid and the trapezium and trapezoid.[83] Imaging with CT helps to identify occult fractures in patients with chronic pain and localized tenderness after trauma to the hand.[86]

Treatment

Closed reduction of trapeziometacarpal dorsal dislocation is performed with longitudinal traction followed by palmar flexion of the wrist, particularly on the second metacarpal, and dorsal pressure on the trapezoid.[83,87] If the reduction is unstable, percutaneous pin fixation is usually sufficient. Fractures involving joint incongruity or irreducible dislocations are best treated with open reduction and pin or screw fixation.[88] Trapezoid excision in fracture dislocation is contraindicated due to the proximal migration of the index metacarpal.[83,85] Hardware is left in place for 6 to 8 weeks. Unrestricted use is permitted by 12 weeks.

Complications

The trapezoid receives 70% of its interosseous supply through dorsal branches.[52,76] Dorsal dislocations disrupting the dorsal blood supply place the trapezoid at risk for AVN.[89] Symptomatic malunions and nonunions can be treated by arthrodesis of the CMC joint.[17]

PISIFORM FRACTURES
Incidence

Despite its prominence at the base of the hypothenar eminence, the pisiform is fractured much less commonly than the hook of hamate, constituting about 1% of carpal fractures.[26] Approximately half of pisiform fractures are associated with other carpal injuries.[17] In isolation, pisiform fractures can be sagittal avulsion fractures, transverse avulsion fractures, or comminuted fractures.[90]

Mechanism of Injury

The anatomy and multiple structures attached to the pisiform play a role in fracture pattern and management. The pisiform articulates with the triquetrum dorsally, is the origin of the abductor digiti minimi, and serves as the attachment for the flexor carpi ulnaris (FCU) that continues distally as the pisohamate and pisometacarpal ligaments. The TCL also attaches to the pisiform. The pisiform forms the radial wall to Guyon's canal, placing the ulnar nerve and artery at risk when fractured.

Pisiform fractures most commonly occur as a result of a direct blow, such as striking the palm during a fall, during a motor vehicle collision, the brunt of a handgun while firing weapons,[20] or racquet sports.[91] Avulsion of the FCU during resisted hyperextension of the wrist can create a transverse fracture pattern.[90] An analogy has been drawn to the patella, whereby direct blows onto the knee often result in comminuted fractures, whereas an avulsion fracture from the patellar tendon results in a transverse fracture pattern.

Pisiform dislocations have been described as a result of blunt trauma and falls on an outstretched wrist.[92–94]

Examination

Point tenderness over the pisiform or during a shuck maneuver of the pisiform should raise suspicion for fracture. Ulnar-sided wrist pain can be replicated with resisted wrist flexion. Ulnar nerve function should be documented.

Radiographic Examination

Standard radiographs can miss all but the large pisiform fractures due to overlying bone. The carpal tunnel view can more easily demonstrate a pisiform fracture. A reverse oblique view with the wrist in 30 degrees of supination places the pisiform on profile (**Fig. 18**). Studies have shown a consistent parallel relation between the pisiform and triquetrum. Pisotriquetral joint injury should be considered if joint separation is greater than 3 mm or bone surfaces are more than 20 degrees from parallel.[95] Imaging with CT is warranted when the results of plain radiography produces an equivocal result.

Treatment

Successful results have been reported when pisiformectomy is properly performed for pisotriquetral arthritis.[96] Hence, when treating athletes with pisiform fractures, the athlete's goal of quick, safe return to sport can be accomplished with early pisiform excision. Cast immobilization for 4 to 6 weeks can be attempted for acute nondisplaced or small avulsion type fractures when time lost from training or participation is not crucial. Widely displaced fractures with decreased FCU function or symptomatic nonunions are best treated with pisiformectomy.[9,17,20,32,46]

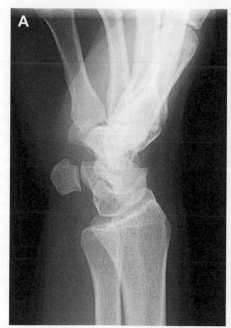

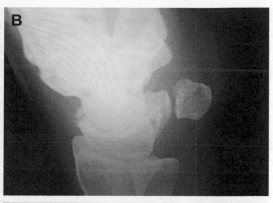

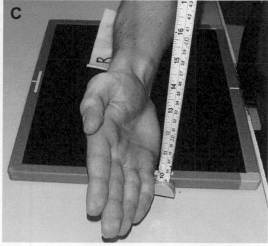

Fig. 18. Semi-supinated carpal radiograph of a normal pisotriquetral joint (*A*) and pisiform fracture (*B*). Proper positioning for the reverse oblique carpal view places the hand in 30-degree supination on the cassette (*C*).

Pisiform excision can be performed through an anterior or lateral approach. The anterior approach is the preferred approach whereby the ulnar nerve is mobilized and gently retracted toward the radial side of the palm. A penetrating towel clip facilitates removal. The pisiform is shaped like a top hat. Care should be taken as the dissection proceeds over the brim of the hat on its radial border. This procedure places the blade close to the ulnar nerve. It is for this reason that the anterior approach is preferred; the lateral approach necessitates a blind release of the bone's radial attachments. Pisiform excision has been performed arthroscopically, but the authors have no personal experience with that technique.

Rehabilitation after pisiform excision is identical to that following excision of a hamate hook, as described earlier. Return to sport is primarily limited by scar sensitivity.

Complications

Ulnar nerve injuries at the time of injury are often neuropraxias[97,98] that resolve with observation.

Cautious monitoring of ulnar nerve deficits is reasonable for 8 to 12 weeks after acute pisiform fracture. Nerve exploration with pisiformectomy is recommended if nerve deficits persist after 12 weeks or worsen at any time during treatment.[17]

Ulnar nerve dysfunction after pisiform excision is common. If the nerve was visualized and protected throughout the procedure, observation is reasonable for 8 to 12 weeks. If the nerve was not visualized, immediate exploration is recommended if the 2-point discrimination is greater than 15 mm or if the patient has developed marked intrinsic weakness.

LUNATE FRACTURES
Incidence

Acute fractures to the lunate are rare, constituting 1% of all carpal fractures.[99] Lunate fractures are classified into 5 subtypes based on the vascularity of the bone and location: volar pole, dorsal pole, transverse body, sagittal body, and osteochondral or chip fractures. The most common subtype is the volar pole fracture.[99]

Mechanism of Injury

The lunate is compressed between the distal radius and capitate with extreme wrist hyperextension and ulnar deviation such as during a fall on an outstretched hand. In sports, lunate fractures have been described following a blow to the hand by a ball in line with the forearm.[100]

Examination

Tenderness over the dorsal aspect of the lunate should raise suspicion of a lunate fracture or scapholunate ligament injury. The pain can be accentuated by wrist motion.

Radiographic Examination

Standard radiographic views can miss a small fracture due to overlying bones. Imaging with CT scan or MRI is indicated if clinical examination suggests an occult fracture or ligament injury (**Fig. 19**).

Treatment

Treatment of athletes with lunate fractures is identical to that of triquetral fractures, as described earlier. Marginal chip fractures are often old injuries discovered as incidental findings in a person with a simple wrist sprain. Treatment is tailored according to pain, swelling, and radiographic findings. Small mariginal chip fractures are treated with short courses of immobilization followed by re-examination and re-imaging. Malalignment of the capitate over the lunate or a scapholunate diastasis is consistent with carpal instability. A volar intercalated segment instability (VISI) deformity with a palmar chip fracture or dorsal intercalated segment instability (DISI) deformity with a dorsal chip necessitates operative fixation. It is worthwhile obtaining contralateral views

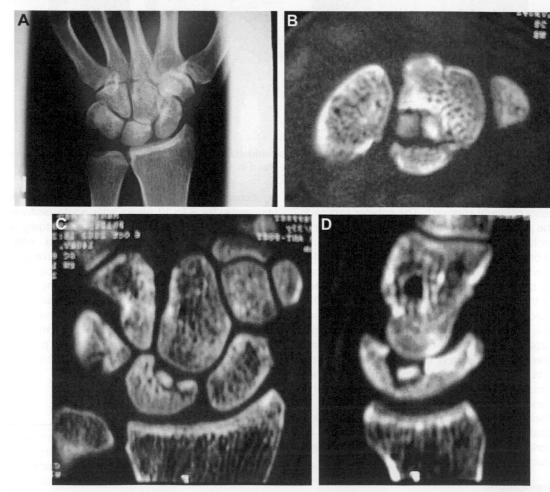

Fig. 19. The curvature of the lunate surfaces and position of the bone in the proximal row can obscure lunate body fractures on standard radiographs (*A*). CT clearly illustrates a lunate body fracture on axial, coronal, and sagittal views (*B–D*).

of the wrist, particularly in a woman with a VISI pattern, as this can be a normal variant.

An extended carpal tunnel approach exposes the volar lunate. Volar pole fractures are often small and may not tolerate headless screw fixation. In those cases the fragment can be secured with a buried pin and a wire suture looped around the volar fibers of the scapholunate ligament.

Fractures that extend into the body of the lunate and into the articular surface are best characterized with CT imaging. The joint surfaces are best seen and reduced through a dorsal approach to the wrist. Comminuted fractures can be managed with cancellous grafting. The construct can be protected with a spanning external fixator.

Complications

Twenty percent of lunates have only a palmar nutrient artery supplying the bone.[52] Displaced volar fragment fractures left untreated place such lunates at risk of AVN and should be anatomically reduced and fixed into place.[101]

There is no consensus on the causal relationship between acute lunate fractures and AVN, or Keinbock disease.[100–102] Long-term follow-up of lunate fractures have failed to show AVN despite half of those patients having ulnar minus variant wrists.[100] There is still reason to be concerned for disruption of the interosseous blood supply with the infrequent horizontal fractures.[102,103] Persistent wrist pain in an athlete following lunate fracture can be evaluated with MR for evidence of AVN. Analyzing the MR for AVN can be difficult. There will be extensive signal change along the lines of fracture. AVN should be diagnosed when there is a homogeneous loss of signal in the entire lunate.

Lunate fractures with intraarticular extension are at risk of midcarpal arthritis.

SUMMARY

Fractures of the carpal bones in athletes are often sport-specific injuries, which can be diagnosed with a complete clinical and radiographic examination of the patient's hand. Special radiographic views can help with the initial assessment; CT and MRI are useful for difficult diagnoses. However, the threshold for obtaining an MRI in an athlete with what seems to be a significant injury is low. The energy imparted on the hand not only creates fractures, but can injure crucial ligaments. Most nondisplaced fractures of the hand can be treated nonoperatively. Early surgical intervention is warranted for displaced intraarticular fractures or carpal malalignment. Excision of the hamate hook and trapezial ridge fractures facilitate an early return to sports.

ACKNOWLEDGMENT

The authors would like to acknowledge Jill Clemente, MS, Research Assistant for her editorial assistance.

REFERENCES

1. Bergfeld JA, Welker GG, Andrish JT, et al. Soft playing splint for protection of significant hand and wrist injuries in sports. Am J Sports Med 1982;10:293–6.
2. DeHaven KE, Lintner DM. Athletic injuries: comparison by age, sport, and gender. Am J Sports Med 1986;14:218–24.
3. Krahl H, Michaelis U, Pieper HG, et al. Stimulation of bone growth through sports: a radiologic investigation of the upper extremities in professional tennis players. Am J Sports Med 1994;22:751–7.
4. Rettig AC, Ryan RO, Stone JA. Epidemiology of hand injuries in sports. In: Strickland JW, Retting AC, editors. Hand injuries in athletes. Philadelphia: WB Saunders; 1992. p. 37–44.
5. Bartone NF, Greico RV. Fractures of the triquetrum. J Bone Joint Surg 1956;38:353–6.
6. Bryan RS, Dobyns JH. Fractures of the carpal bones other than the lunate and navicular. Clin Orthop Relat Res 1980;14:107–11.
7. Hocker K, Menschik A. Chip fractures of the triquetrum. J Hand Surg Br 1994;19:584–8.
8. Bonnin JG, Greening WP. Fractures of the triquetrum. Br J Surg 1944;31:278–83.
9. Botte MJ, Gelberman RH. Fractures of the carpus, excluding the scaphoid. Hand Clin 1987;3(1):149–61.
10. Cohen MS. Fractures of the carpal bones. Hand Clin 1997;13(4):587–99.
11. DeBeer JD, Hudson DA. Fractures of the triquetrum. J Hand Surg Br 1987;12:52–3.
12. Greening WP. Isolated fracture of the carpal cuneiform. Br Med J 1942;1:221–2.
13. Fairbank TJ. Chip fractures of the os triquetrum. Br Med J 1942;2:310–1.
14. Levy M, Fischel RE, Stern GM, et al. Chip fractures of the os triquetrum. The mechanism of injury. J Bone Joint Surg Br 1979;61:355–7.
15. Garcia-Elias M. Dorsal fractures of the triquetrum—avulsion or compression fractures? J Hand Surg Am 1987;12:266–8.
16. Mayfield JK, Johnson RB, Kilcoyne RK. Carpal dislocations: pathomechanics and progressive perilunar instability. J Hand Surg Am 1980;5:226–41.
17. Vigler M, Aviles A, Lee SK. Carpal fractures excluding the scaphoid. Hand Clin 2006;22:501–16.

18. Culp RW, Lemel M, Taras JS. Complications of common carpal injuries. Hand Clin 1994;10(1): 139–55.

19. Papp S. Carpal bone fractures. Orthop Clin North Am 2007;38:251–60.

20. Geissler WB. Carpal fractures in athletes. Clin Sports Med 2001;20(1):167–88.

21. Porter ML, Seehra K. Fracture-dislocation of the triquetrum treated with a Herbert screw. J Bone Joint Surg Br 1991;73:347–8.

22. Suzuki T, Nakatsuchi Y, Tatweiwa Y, et al. Osteochondral fracture of the triquetrum: a case report. J Hand Surg Am 2002;27:98–100.

23. Aiki H, Wada T, Yamashita T. Pisotriquetral arthrosis after triquetral malunion: a case report. J Hand Surg Am 2006;31:1157–9.

24. Garcia-Elias M. Carpal bone fractures (excluding scaphoid fractures). In: Watson HK, Weinberg J, editors. The wrist. Philadelphia: Lippincott Williams & Wilkins; 2001. p. 174–81.

25. Walsh JJ, Bishop AT. Diagnosis and management of hamate hook fractures. Hand Clin 2000;16(3): 397–403.

26. Boulas HJ, Milek MA. Hook of the hamate fractures. Orthop Rev 1990;19(6):518–22.

27. Polivy KD, Millender LH, Newberg A, et al. Fractures of the hook of the hamate—a failure of clinical diagnosis. J Hand Surg Am 1985;10:101–4.

28. Thomas AP, Birch. An unusual hamate fracture. Hand 1983;3:281–6.

29. Hirano K, Inoue G. Classification and treatment of hamate fractures. Hand Surg 2005;10:151–7.

30. Chase JM, Light TR, Benson LS. Coronal fracture of the hamate body. Am J Orthop 1997;26(8): 568–71.

31. Bishop AT, Beckenbaugh RD. Fracture of the hamate hook. J Hand Surg Am 1988;13:135–9.

32. Rettig AC. Athletic injuries of the wrist and hand: part I: traumatic injuries of the wrist. Am J Sports Med 2003;31:1038–48.

33. Manske PR. Fracture of the hook of the hamate presenting as carpal tunnel syndrome. Hand 1978;10: 181–3.

34. Foucher G, Schuind F, Merle M, et al. Fractures of the hook of the hamate. J Hand Surg Br 1985;10: 205–10.

35. Cameron HU, Hastings DE, Fournasier VL. Fracture of the hook of the hamate.A case report. J Bone Joint Surg Am 1975;57:276–7.

36. Norman A, Nelson J, Green S. Fractures of the hook of hamate: radiographic signs. Radiology 1985;154:49–53.

37. Hart VL, Gaynor V. Roentgenographic study of the carpal canal. J Bone Joint Surg Am 1941; 23:382–3.

38. Andress MR, Peckar VG. Fracture of the hook of the hamate. Br J Radiol 1970;43:141–3.

39. Stark HH, Jobe FW, Boyes JH, et al. Fracture of the hook of hamate in athletes. J Bone Joint Surg Am 1977;59:575–82.

40. Papilion JD, Dupuy TE, Aulicino PL, et al. Radiographic evaluation of the hook of the hamate: a new technique. J Hand Surg Am 1988;13:437–9.

41. Andresen R, Radmer S, Sparmann M, et al. Imaging of hamate bone fractures in conventional X-rays and high-resolution computed tomography: an in vitro study. Invest Radiol 1999;34:46–50.

42. Kato H, Nakamura R, Horii E, et al. Diagnostic imaging for fracture of the hook of the hamate. Hand Surg 2000;5(1):19–24.

43. Freeland AE, Finley JS. Displaced dorsal oblique fracture of the hamate treated with a cortical mini lag screw. J Hand Surg Am 1986;11:656–8.

44. Whalen JL, Bishop AT, Linscheid RL. Nonoperative treatment of acute hamate hook fractures. J Hand Surg Am 1992;17:507–11.

45. Carroll RE, Lakin JF. Fracture of the hook of the hamate: acute treatment. J Trauma 1993;34(6):803–5.

46. Rettig ME, Dassa GL, Raskin KB, et al. Distal radius and carpal fractures. Clin Sports Med 1998;17(3): 469–89.

47. Demirkan F, Calandruccio JH, DiAngelo D. Biomechanical evaluation of flexor tendon function after hamate hook excision. J Hand Surg Am 2003;28: 138–43.

48. Scheuffler O, Andresen R, Radmer S, et al. Hook of hamate fractures: critical evaluation of different therapeutic procedures. Plast Reconstr Surg 2005;115:488–97.

49. Konig PS, Hage JJ, Bloem JJ, et al. Variations of the ulnar nerve and ulnar artery in Guyon's canal: a cadaveric study. J Hand Surg Am 1994;19:617–22.

50. Ahsoh K, Kondo M, Torisu T, et al. The lateral approach compared with the volar approach for exposure of the hook of the hamate. Clin Orthop Relat Res 1989;239:217–21.

51. Aldridge JM, Mallon WJ. Hook of the hamate fractures in competitive golfers: results of treatment by excision of the fractured hook of the hamate. Orthopedics 2003;26:717–9.

52. Panagis JS, Gelberman RH, Taleisnik J, et al. The arterial anatomy of the human carpus. Part II: the intraosseous vascularity. J Hand Surg Am 1983; 8(4):375–82.

53. Failla JM. Hook of hamate vascularity: vulnerability to osteonecrosis and nonunion. J Hand Surg Am 1993;18:1075–9.

54. Van Demark RE, Parke WW. Avascular necrosis of the hamate: a case report with reference to the hamate blood supply. J Hand Surg Am 1992;17: 1086–90.

55. Failla JM. Osteonecrosis associated with nonunion of the hook of the hamate. Orthopedics 1993;16(2): 217–8.

56. Smith P, Wright TW, Wallace PF, et al. Excision of the hook of the hamate: a retrospective survey and review of the literature. J Hand Surg Br 1988; 13:612–5.

57. Garcia-Elias M, Henriquez-Lluch A, Rossignani P, et al. Bennett's fracture combined with fracture of the trapezium. A report of three cases. J Hand Surg Br 1993;18:523–6.

58. Cordrey LJ, Ferror-Torrells M. Management of fractures of the greater multangular. J Bone Joint Surg Am 1960;42:1111–8.

59. Palmer AK. Trapezial ridge fractures. J Hand Surg Am 1981;6:561–4.

60. Walker JL, Greene TL, Lunseth PA. Fractures of the body of the trapezium. J Orthop Trauma 1988;2: 22–8.

61. McGuigan FX, Culp RW. Surgical treatment of intra-articular fractures of the trapezium. J Hand Surg Am 2002;27:697–703.

62. Pointu J, Schwenck JP, Destree G, et al. Fractures of the trapezium. Mechanism, pathology and indications for treatment. French J Orthop Surg 1988; 2:380–91.

63. McClain EJ, Boyes JH. Missed fractures of the greater multangular. J Bone Joint Surg Am 1966; 48:1525–8.

64. Binhammer P, Born T. Coronal fracture of the body of the trapezium. A case report. J Hand Surg Am 1998;23:156–7.

65. Checroun AJ, Mekhail AO, Ebraheim NA. Radial artery injury in association with fractures of the trapezium. J Hand Surg Br 1997;22:419–22.

66. Gelberman RH, Vance RM, Zakaib GS. Fractures at the base of the thumb: treatment with oblique traction. J Bone Joint Surg Am 1979;61:260–2.

67. Botte MJ, von Schroeder HP, Gellman H, et al. Fracture of the trapezial ridge. Clin Orthop Relat Res 1992;276:202–5.

68. Rand JA, Linscheid RL, Dobyns JH. Capitate fractures: a long-term follow-up. Clin Orthop Relat Res 1982;165:209–16.

69. Fenton RL. The naviculo-capitate fracture syndrome. J Bone Joint Surg Am 1956;38:681–4.

70. Vance RM, Gelberman RH, Evans EF. Scaphocapitate fractures. Patterns of dislocation, mechanisms of injury, and preliminary results of treatment. J Bone Joint Surg 1980;62:271–6.

71. Stein F, Seigel MW. Naviculocapitate fracture syndrome. A case report: new thought on mechanism of injury. J Bone Joint Surg Am 1969;51:391–5.

72. Volk AG, Schnall SB, Merkle P, et al. Unusual capitate fracture: a case report. J Hand Surg Am 1995; 20:581–2.

73. Albertsen J, Mencke S, Christensen L, et al. Isolated capitate fracture diagnosed by computed tomography. Case report. Mandchir Mikrochir Plast Chir 1999;31:79–81.

74. Calandruccio JH, Duncan SF. Isolated non-displaced capitate waist fracture diagnosed by magnetic resonance imaging. J Hand Surg Am 1999;24:856–9.

75. Richards RR, Paitich B, Bell RS. Internal fixation of a capitate fracture with Hebert screws. J Hand Surg Am 1990;15:885–7.

76. Gelberman RH, Panagis JS, Taleisnik, et al. The arterial anatomy of the human carpus. Part I: the extraosseous vascularity. J Hand Surg Am 1983; 8:367–75.

77. Vander Grend R, Dell PC, Glowczewskie F, et al. Intraosseous blood supply of the capitate and its correlation with aseptic necrosis. J Hand Surg Am 1984;9:677–80.

78. Lowry WE, Cord SA. Traumatic avascular necrosis of the capitate bone-case report. J Hand Surg Am 1981;6:245–8.

79. Kimmel RB, O'Brien ET. Surgical treatment of avascular necrosis of the proximal pole of the capitate-case report. J Hand Surg Am 1982;7:284–6.

80. Lapinsky AS, Mack GR. Avascular necrosis of the capitate: a case report. J Hand Surg Am 1992;17: 1090–2.

81. Adler JB, Shaftan GW. Fractures of the capitate. J Bone Joint Surg Am 1962;44:1537–47.

82. Rico AA, Holguin PH, Martin JG. Peudoarthrosis of the capitate. J Hand Surg Br 1999;24:382–4.

83. Stein AH. Dorsal dislocation of the lesser multangular bone. J Bone Joint Surg Am 1971;53: 377–9.

84. Garcia-Elias M, Dobyns JM, Cooney WP, et al. Traumatic dislocations of the carpus. J Hand Surg Am 1989;14:446–57.

85. Lewis HH. Dislocation of the lesser multangular. J Bone Joint Surg Am 1962;44:1412–4.

86. Nagumo A, Toh S, Tsubo K, et al. An occult fracture of the trapezoid bone. J Bone Joint Surg Am 2002; 84:1025–6.

87. Meyn MA, Roth AM. Isolated dislocation of the trapezoid bone. J Hand Surg Am 1980;5:602–4.

88. Yasuwaki Y, Nagata Y, Yamamoto T, et al. J Hand Surg Am 1994;19:457–9.

89. Cuenod P, Della Santa DR. Open dislocation of the trapezoid. J Hand Surg Br 1995;20:185–8.

90. Patel MM, Catalano LW. Carpal fractures excluding the scaphoid. In: Trumble TE, Budoff JE, editors. Hand surgery update IV. Rosemont (IL): American Society for Surgery of the Hand; 2007. p. 259–70.

91. Helal B. Racquet player's pisiform. Hand 1978;10: 87–90.

92. Immerman EW. Dislocation of the pisiform. J Bone Joint Surg Am 1948;30:489–92.

93. Muniz AE. Unusual wrist pain: pisiform dislocation and fracture. J Emerg Med 1999;17(3):469–89.

94. Fleege MA, Jebson PJ, Renfrew DL, et al. Pisiform fractures. Skeletal Radiol 1991;20:169–72.

95. Vasilas A, Greico RV, Bartone NF. Roentgen aspects of injuries to the pisiform bone and pisotriquetral joint. J Bone Joint Surg Am 1960;42:1317–28.

96. Carroll RE, Coyle MP. Dysfunction of the pisotriquetral joint: treatment by excision of the pisiform. J Hand Surg Am 1985;10:703–7.

97. Israeli A, Engel J, Ganel A. Possible fatigue fracture of the pisiform bone in volleyball players. Int J Sports Med 1982;3:56–7.

98. Matsunaga D, Uchiyama S, Nakagawa H, et al. Lower ulnar nerve palsy related to fracture of the pisiform bone in patients with multiple injuries. J Trauma 2002;53:364–8.

99. Teisen H, Hjarbaek J. Classification of fresh fractures of the lunate. J Hand Surg Br 1988;13:458–62.

100. Teisen H, Hjarbaek J, Jensen EK. Follow-up investigation of fresh lunate bone fracture. Handchir Mikrochir Plast Chir 1990;22:20–2.

101. Freeland AE, Ahmad N. Oblique shear fractures of the lunate. Orthopedics 2003;26:806–8.

102. Beckenbaugh RD, Shives TC, Dobyns JH, et al. Kienbock's disease: the natural history of Kienbock's disease and consideration of lunate fractures. Clin Orthop 1980;149:98–106.

103. Gelberman RH, Bauman TD, Menton J, et al. The vascularity of the lunate bone and Kienbock's disease. J Hand Surg Am 1980;5:272–8.

Repair of Arthroscopic Triangular Fibrocartilage Complex Tears in Athletes

Periklis A. Papapetropoulos, MD[a,b], David S. Ruch, MD[a,b,*]

KEYWORDS

- Triangular fibrocartilage complex repair
- Arthroscopic • Athletes • Wrist injury • Wrist stability

Triangular fibrocartilage complex (TFCC) is an important stabilizer and load absorber of the wrist. Injuries of the TFCC can result in wrist pain that prohibits performance in athletes. The most common injury is wrist rotation; a fall on the extended-pronated wrist or traction is frequently reported. The complaints may be vague and include ulnar-sided pain, which may be associated with a palpable click with forearm rotation. Examination typically reveals point tenderness at the fovea of wrist between the extensor carpi ulnaris (ECU) and the flexor carpi ulnaris (FCU) distal to the ulnar head. Treatment options typically start with conservative measures including wrist splints, injections, and iontophoresis. When the patients have exhausted conservative measures, operative treatment may be considered. Operative measures include open or arthroscopic repair, debridement, or ulnar shortening osteotomy.[1–4] This article describes the surgical management and results of treatment of TFCC injuries in athletes.

In a follow-up study of 25 patients with TFCC tear and ulnar positive variance, Minami and Kato[5] found that ulnar shortening resulted in relief of symptoms in 23 of 25 patients. Westkaemper[6] noted that in patients with TFCC tears, the results were poor in the presence of an associated lunotriquetral ligament tear. Trumble and colleagues[7] noted poor results after TFCC repair with ulnar positive variance, and recommended a combined approach of triangular fibrocartilage complex repair with subsequent ulnar shortening osteotomy. Arthroscopy can be particularly valuable to the surgeon because it can be used as a diagnostic tool that also enables treatment of the tears.[8,9] Among the various methods of treatment, arthroscopically assisted repair remains attractive to physicians and patients because of the minimal injury related to the surgery and the short recovery time, especially useful for the high demands of professional athletes. Therefore, although the arthroscopic procedure may be technically demanding, studies indicate that repair using an arthroscopic approach provides relief of symptoms in most patients.[10–14]

Treating athletes with TFCC injuries can be difficult. Each athlete has individual priorities and concerns, ranging from general health and fitness for the recreational athlete to earning or potentially earning a living as a professional.[15,16] It is crucial for the treating surgeon to understand these issues and to offer the appropriate treatment options at the appropriate time. The goal of the treatment of the competitive athlete with TFCC tear is to obtain maximal recovery and return to

The authors did not receive any outside funding or grants in support of their research for or preparation of this work.

a Hand, Upper Extremity and Microvascular Surgery Fellowship Training Program, Department of Surgery, Division of Orthopaedic Surgery, Duke University Medical Center, Trent Drive, Durham, NC 27710, USA
b Division of Orthopaedic Surgery, Department of Surgery, Duke University Medical Center, Hospital South, Orange Zone, 5FT Floor, Room 5332, Trent Drive, Durham, NC 27710, USA
* Corresponding author. Division of Orthopaedic Surgery, Duke University Medical Center, Hospital South, Orange Zone, 5FT Floor, Room 5332, Trent Drive, Durham, NC, 27710.
E-mail address: d.ruch@duke.edu (D.S. Ruch).

Hand Clin 25 (2009) 389–394
doi:10.1016/j.hcl.2009.05.011

the preinjury level of performance. Early wrist arthroscopy and treatment of TFCC pathology in this population is certainly a real and valuable treatment option.

MATERIALS AND METHODS

From 1995 to 2007, the author has performed 25 arthroscopic procedures on the wrist in professional athletes. All 25 wrists had negative or neutral ulnar variance. Fourteen professional tennis players and 11 golf players underwent arthroscopic TFCC repairs by a single surgeon who used the same technique. The preoperative assessment, surgical technique, and preliminary results are presented in this article.

Preoperative Evaluation

Preoperative assessment consists of characteristic history, symptoms, findings of pertinent examinations, and imaging assessment. Patients sustained a supination injury with or without axial load. Patients reported painful click with supination movements, burning dysesthesias at the ulnocarpal joint, and pain with tight grasp. Physical findings include point tenderness at the interval between the ECU/FCU tendons immediately distal to the ulnar head, and pain with attempted carpal supination on the fixed ulna relative to the radius. Less frequent findings include a positive ulnar impaction test (ulnar deviation and axial load) and a positive lunotriquetral shear test.

Imaging Findings

The evaluation of ulnar-sided wrist pain remains controversial. Arthrography has been demonstrated to have a false-negative rate of up to 50%. MRI has significant false negatives because of granulation at the periphery of the disk, making the test useful for central tears but less reliable for peripheral tears. MRI arthrography is useful in defining central perforations but less useful in defining peripheral TFCC lesions (**Fig. 1**).

Operative Indications

Arthroscopic evaluation and possible TFCC debridement or repair is indicated when the patient has failed 4 months of nonoperative management, has ulnar-sided wrist pain resulting in a significant decrease in grip strength (less than 80% of the contralateral side), and whose radiographs, including a pronated grip view, do not demonstrate evidence of ulnar impaction syndrome.

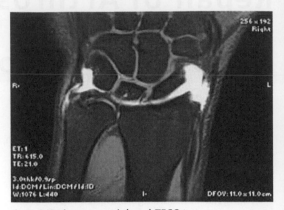

Fig. 1. MRI image: peripheral TFCC tear.

Arthroscopic Evaluation

Evaluation of ulnar-sided wrist pain includes thorough evaluation of the radiocarpal joints. Focus is addressed on the lunotriquetral ligament and the chondral surfaces of the lunate and triquetrum. If a peripheral tear is identified (**Figs. 2** and **3**) a shaver is placed in the 6-R portal, and any synovitis and granulation tissue must be debrided. A probe then is inserted and the stability of the articular disc is evaluated (**Figs. 4** and **5**).

Indication for repair rather than a debridement includes a peripheral tear involving 50% or more of the articular disk-capsular insertion, ulnar neutral or ulnar negative variance, and the absence of associated injuries that would indicate the need for ulnar shortening osteotomy. Contraindications include those factors that would predispose the surgeon to perform an ulnar shortening

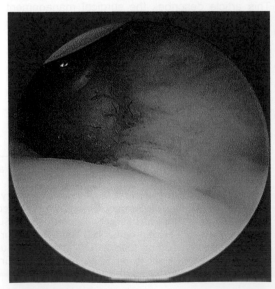

Fig. 2. Peripheral TFCC tear.

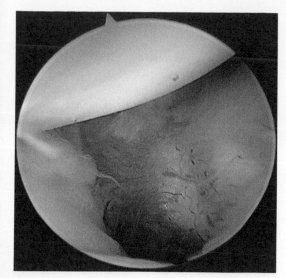

Fig. 3. Peripheral TFCC tear.

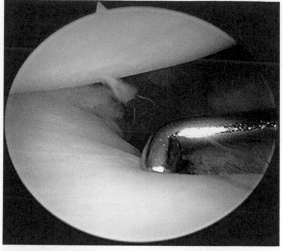

Fig. 5. Evaluation of TFCC stability.

osteotomy. Specific findings that predispose to osteotomy rather than repair include ulnar positive variance of 2 mm on a pronated grip view, complete lunotriquetral interosseous ligament tear, and osteochondral lesions of the lunate.

Operative Technique

The arthroscopy is performed using a wrist traction tower for distraction of the wrist. Five to 10 pounds (2.27 to 5.53 kg) of traction are applied. A small joint arthroscope (2.5 mm) with 30-degree viewing field and a small joint debrider are used for synovectomies and for the preparation of the reattachment site of the TFCC (**Fig. 6**).

The operative technique in the series is an arthroscopic repair of the peripheral margin of the avulsed articular disk back to the capsule and the ECU subsheath using three 2-0 polydioxanone (PDS) sutures placed under arthroscopic visualization. The dorsal two sutures are placed to the ECU subsheath by using a meniscal needle repair technique with a Touhy needle.

Repair of the TFCC is performed with the arthroscope in the 3-4 or 4-5 portal (**Fig. 6**). The 3-4 portal is preferred because it provides a better perspective of the entire ulnar side of the wrist. The surgeon may find it useful to maintain a probe in the 4-5 or 6-R portals. This probe is useful in the manipulation of the repair needles (see **Figs. 4** and **5**).

A 1-cm incision is made at the 6-R interval, and careful identification of the branches of the dorsal sensory portion of the ulnar nerve is performed. Up to 50% of the retinaculum over the ECU is incised

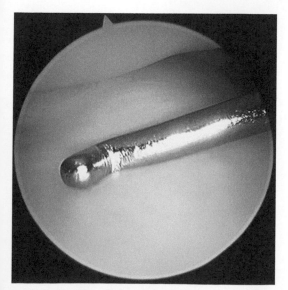

Fig. 4. Evaluation of TFCC stability.

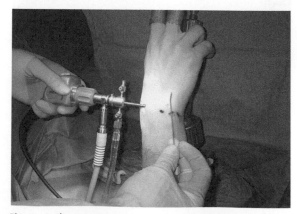

Fig. 6. Arthroscope, portals, and needle.

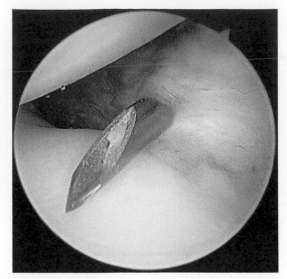

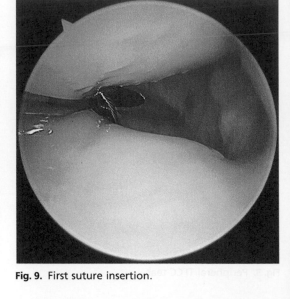

Fig. 7. Needle insertion.

Fig. 9. First suture insertion.

and the tendon then may be retracted radially and ulnarly.

The curved needle from a meniscus repair set (Smith & Nephew, Memphis, Tennessee) (see **Fig. 6**) or a TFCC repair kit (Linvatec) then may be inserted at the radial margin of the ECU subsheath and passed through the peripheral edge of the articular disc (**Fig. 7**). A straight needle then may be inserted 1 cm distal to the first needle.

A wire snare is inserted (usually through the curved needle), and the end of the straight needle is captured (**Fig. 8**). A 2-0 polydioxanone (PDS) suture is then passed through the straight needle, advancing as much suture as possible into the joint (**Figs. 9** and **10**).

The curved needle and snare subsequently are withdrawn, also pulling the suture out. A second suture is then placed at the ulnar aspect of the ECU subsheath (**Fig. 11**). Finally, stabilization is achieved with three sutures (**Fig. 12**). Irritation of the ECU may be minimized by not placing these sutures directly below the tendon.

Palmar-sided tears may be addressed by using this same technique; however, a second incision may be required to ensure that injury does not occur to the ulnar artery or ulnar nerve. A second technique of placement of palmar-sided sutures may be performed using the Touhy needle. This blunt-tipped needle is used by anesthesiologists for the placement of epidural catheters. The

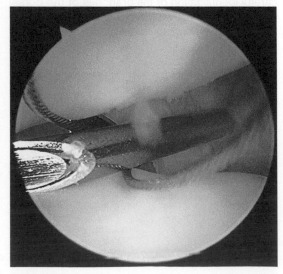

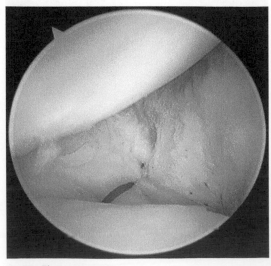

Fig. 8. Wire snare.

Fig. 10. First suture.

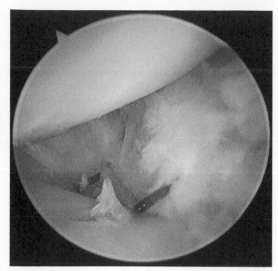

Fig. 11. Sutures.

needle is introduced through the 1-2 portal and passed through the radiocarpal joint to pass through the peripheral ulnar portion of the TFCC and out of the palmar side of the wrist. The trocar then can be withdrawn, and a 2-0 polydioxanone suture (PDS) can be advanced. A hemostat then may be placed on the radial joint, and a second pass made from cutting the protruding suture. The radial hemostat is removed, and both ends of the suture are brought out of the ulnar side of the wrist. An incision is made between the two sutures and dissection is performed down to the level of the capsule. Care is taken to avoid trapping the transverse articular branches of the dorsal nerve.

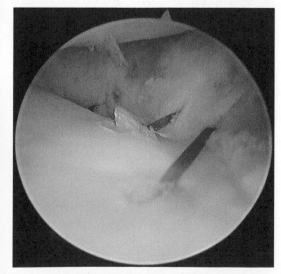

Fig. 12. Final arthroscopic image of TFCC sutures.

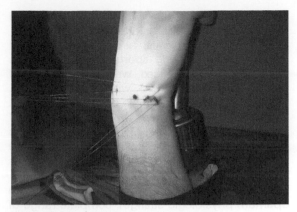

Fig. 13. Suture knots.

The sutures then are tied with the wrist in supination and ulnar deviation. They are tied down over the ulnar-sided capsule, and the arthroscope can confirm obliteration of the tear. Alternatively, the sutures may be tied over a button to avoid prominence of the knot in the subcutaneous tissue at the ulnar side of the wrist (**Fig. 13**).

POSTOPERATIVE COURSE

Postoperatively, the patients are maintained in a sugar splint or cast in 60 degrees of supination for 3.5 weeks. Range of motion then is initiated to neutral rotation and neutral deviation. Full pronation is not encouraged until 5 weeks postoperatively. At 6 weeks, strong grip and full range of motion are expected.

COMPLICATIONS

True complications of this procedure are uncommon but include entrapment of the transverse branch of the dorsal sensory branch of the ulnar nerve, irritation of the ECU or sensory nerve by the presence of the suture knot, or loss of full pronation. Attention must always be paid to the small sensory branches of the ulnar nerve. There were no complications in the present series.

SUMMARY

The hand and wrist are the most active portion of the upper extremity, are the least well protected, and are therefore at high risk for injury during sports activity.[17] These injuries can be caused by repeated loads or following a specific traumatic event.[18] Hand and wrist injuries are common in athletes, accounting for up to 15% of all sports injuries.[19,20] Wrist injuries in the athlete constitute a unique orthopedic challenge. Because of the particular demands on the athlete (eg, financial implications, coaching and administration pressures, self-esteem issues), a specialized management approach is often necessary.[21]

In the present series, all patients sustained a TFCC injury during sports activity. Patients present with ulnar-sided wrist pain, some of them with a palpable click with forearm rotation. Physical examination reveals point tenderness at the fovea of wrist between the ECU and the FCU distal to the ulnar head. MRI was performed to confirm and reveal the side and extent of the TFCC injury. After the establishment of diagnosis all patients were treated arthroscopically.

In conclusion, in high-demand athletes, in whom optimum physiologic strength, complete range of motion, stability, and the shortest possible postoperative period and bone-healing process after ulna shortening, without large skin incisions, are essential, the arthroscopic repair of TFCC tears is becoming the treatment of choice.

REFERENCES

1. Boulas HJ, Milek MA. Ulnar shortening for tears of the triangular fibrocartilaginous complex. J Hand Surg Am 1990;15(3):415–20.

2. Cerofolini E, Luchetti R, Perzini L, et al. MR evaluation of triangular fibrocartilage complex tears in the wrist: comparison with arthrography and arthroscopy. J Comput Assist Tomogr 1990;14(6):963–7.

3. Hermansdorfer JD, Kleinman WB. Management of chronic peripheral tears of the triangular fibrocartilage complex. J Hand Surg Am 1991;16(2):340–6.

4. Minami A, Ishikawa J, Suenaga N, et al. Clinical results of treatment of triangular fibrocartilage complex tears by arthroscopic debridement. J Hand Surg Am 1996;21(3):406–11.

5. Minami A, Kato H. Ulnar shortening for triangular fibrocartilage complex tears associated with ulnar positive variance. J Hand Surg Am 1998;23(5):904–8.

6. Westkaemper JG, Mitsionis G, Giannakopoulos P, et al. Wrist arthroscopy for the treatment of ligament and triangular fibrocartilage complex injuries. Arthroscopy 1998;14(5):479–83.

7. Trumble TE, Gilbert M, Vedder N, et al. Ulnar shortening combined with arthroscopic repairs in the delayed management of triangular fibrocartilage complex tears. J Hand Surg Am 1997;22(5):807–13.

8. Pederzini L, Luchetti R, Soragni O, et al. Evaluation of the triangular fibrocartilage complex tears by arthroscopy, arthrography, and magnetic resonance imaging. Arthroscopy 1992;8(2):191–7.

9. Peterson JJ, Bancroft LW. Injuries of the fingers and thumb in the athlete. Clin Sports Med 2006;25(3): 527–42, vii–viii.

10. Bednar JM, Osterman AL. The role of arthroscopy in the treatment of traumatic triangular fibrocartilage injuries. Hand Clin 1994;10(4):605–14.

11. Roth JH, Poehling GG. Arthroscopic "-ectomy" surgery of the wrist. Arthroscopy 1990;6(2):141–7.

12. Ruch DS, Papadonikolakis A. Arthroscopically assisted repair of peripheral triangular fibrocartilage complex tears: factors affecting outcome. Arthroscopy 2005;21(9):1126–30.

13. Ruch DS, Ritter MR. Repair of peripheral triangular fibrocartilage complex tears. Atlas Hand Clin 2001; 6(2):211–20.

14. Sagerman SD, Short W. Arthroscopic repair of radial-sided triangular fibrocartilage complex tears. Arthroscopy 1996;12(3):339–42.

15. Dailey SW, Palmer AK. The role of arthroscopy in the evaluation and treatment of triangular fibrocartilage complex injuries in athletes. Hand Clin 2000;16(3): 461–76.

16. Estrella EP, Hung LK, Ho PC, et al. Arthroscopic repair of triangular fibrocartilage complex tears. Arthroscopy 2007;23(7):729–37, 737 e1.

17. Patel D, Dean C, Baker RJ, et al. The hand in sports: an update on the clinical anatomy and physical examination. Prim Care 2005;32(1):71–89.

18. Koh J, Dietz J. Osteoarthritis in other joints (hip, elbow, foot, ankle, toes, wrist) after sports injuries. Clin Sports Med 2005;24(1):57–70.

19. Rettig AC. Epidemiology of hand and wrist injuries in sports. Clin Sports Med 1998;17(3):401–6.

20. Ritter MR, Chang DS, Ruch DS, et al. The role of arthroscopy in the treatment of lunotriquetral ligament injuries. Hand Clin 1999;15(3):445–54, viii.

21. Morgan WJ, Slowman LS. Acute hand and wrist injuries in athletes: evaluation and management. J Am Acad Orthop Surg 2001;9(6):389–400.

Management of Carpal Instability in Athletes

Joseph F. Slade III, MD*, Matthew D. Milewski, MD

KEYWORDS

- Carpal instability • Scaphoid • Carpal fractures
- Biomechanics • Athletics

Hand and wrist injuries are common in most athletic events and sports. The estimated incidence of hand and wrist injuries in athletics constitutes 3% to 9% of all athletic injuries.[1] In particular, wrist injuries in athletes can lead to loss of playing time, inability to perform at preinjury levels, and possible termination of a prospective career.[2] Collision sports such as football have up to 15% of injuries involving the wrist (**Fig. 1**). However, noncontact sports, such as gymnastics, can also have a high incidence of wrist injuries, ranging from 46% to 87% of participants.[3] A recent review of 870 prospective professional football offensive linemen evaluated at the National Football League combine found 18 players had a history of carpal fractures with a range of severity and treatment modalities.[4] Carpal fractures, ligament injury, and resulting carpal instability represent a spectrum of injuries to the wrist in the athletic patient, both in the acute traumatic setting and in the more chronic overuse syndromes.

ANATOMY

The carpus is a complex set of eight bones and connecting ligaments that link the forearm to the hand. The distal row consists of the trapezium, trapezoid, capitate and hamate from radial to ulnar. The proximal row consists of the scaphoid, lunate and triquetrum. The pisiform is a sesamoid bone within the flexor carpi ulnaris tendon at the level of the triquetrum. The scaphoid represents the link between the proximal and distal rows. Extrinsic ligaments are extracapsular and link the distal metacarpals and proximal forearm bones to the carpus. The intrinsic

ligaments are intracapsular and link adjacent carpal bones.[5–7] The lunate is connected to the triquetrum and scaphoid by strong interosseous ligaments. Disruption of these ligaments can lead to dissociative carpal instability.[8] Non-dissociative carpal instability refers to disruption of the extrinsic ligaments and results in instability between the carpal rows or between the radiocarpal joint.

With the scaphoid being a key link between the proximal and distal rows, it is important to consider its specific anatomy. Approximately 80% of the scaphoid is covered by cartilage which limits ligament fixation and vascular channels.[2] Injection studies have confirmed the limited blood supply of the scaphoid with retrograde supply from the radial artery branches through the distal pole.[9] The dorsal radial artery branch enters the scaphoid through the dorsal ridge and provides 70% to 80% of the intraosseous blood supply with the volar branch supply limited to the distal scaphoid tuberosity. This dorsal branch supplies the proximal pole and 20% to 30% of the distal pole. Ninety-three percent of dorsal radial artery branches perforate distal to the waist of the scaphoid. Hence, fractures proximal to the waist of the scaphoid can disrupt endosteal blood supply to the proximal pole.

BIOMECHANICS

The biomechanics of the carpus is complex because of the multitude of bones linked to provide a wide range of motion for positioning of the hand while providing a stable connection between forearm and hand for weight bearing.

Department of Orthopeadics and Rehabilitation, Yale University School of Medicine, PO Box 208071, New Haven, CT 060-8071, USA
* Corresponding author.
E-mail address: joseph.slade@yale.edu (J.F. Slade III).

Hand Clin 25 (2009) 395–408
doi:10.1016/j.hcl.2009.05.002

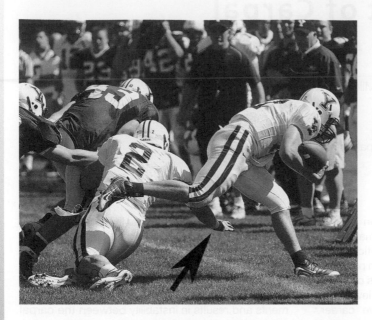

Fig. 1. Collision sports such as football have a significant number of injuries involving the wrist. Injuries can occur from a fall on an outstretched wrist or from direct collision. Carpal fractures or ligament injuries are common in youth because the radius has a high density and resists fractures. (*Courtesy of* Steven Conn, BA and Sam Rubin, BA, New Haven, CT; with permission from Yale Athletics.)

This is particularly important in the athlete whose events will put additional stress and strain across the wrist and will often require the upper extremity to become a weight-bearing limb as in gymnastics. The distal row of the carpus has minimal interosseous motion and works as a unit with the second and third metacarpal bones.[10,11] The proximal row has no direct tendon attachments and has more significant interosseous motion. The scaphoid tends to flex especially with radially deviation to accommodate the trapezium and capitate of the distal row. In contrast, the triquetrum tends to extend because of its helicoid articulation with the hamate.[8] The lunate is balanced in between these two carpal bones by the scapholunate interosseous ligament (SLIL) and lunotriquetral interosseous ligament (LTIL). Disruption of the SLIL will allow the lunate to extend through the pull of triquetrum and the LTIL with the resulting dorsal intercalated segment instability (DISI) pattern. Fracture of the scaphoid can also disrupt this linkage and allow for the extension of the lunate and resultant DISI deformity. Likewise, disruption of the LTIL will allow the lunate to flex with the scaphoid with the resulting volar intercalated segment instability pattern.

In one theory of carpal biomechanics, the scaphoid is believed to be the cross-link or tie-rod linking the proximal and distal rows.[12] In general, approximately 80% of axial joint compressive force is transmitted across radioscaphoid and radiolunate articulations whereas 20% is transmitted by the ulnocarpal joint.[13] Across the radiocarpal joint, 60% of the axial force is believed to be transmitted through the scaphoid fossa and 40% through the

lunate fossa.[14] The mechanisms of injury to the scaphoid and the carpus in general have been studied in detail in several cadaveric studies. The primary requirement appears to be a hyperextension injury past 95°.[15] A fracture of the scaphoid usually begins at the volar waist with a tensile failure then forces propagate to the dorsal surface with compression loading until failure.[16] In another cadaveric study in which the wrists were loaded in extension, ulnar deviation and carpal supination, the scaphoid fractured through the waist as it impinged on the dorsal rim of the radius.[17] Mayfield and colleagues[18] also found that this same mechanism of extension, ulnar deviation and carpal supination produced a progressive perilunar instability pattern. Stage I is characterized by scapholunate diastasis or scaphoid fracture. Increased loading produces stage II with dorsal dislocation of the capitate. Stage III is characterized by lunotriquetral diastasis. Finally, stage IV has complete dislocation of the lunate. Although these studies confirm the usual patterns of injury to the scaphoid and carpal ligaments, flexion injuries to the wrist can also produce scaphoid fractures and should be considered when evaluating the injured athlete's wrist.[8]

The high rate of nonunion that is seen with displaced scaphoid fractures relates to its poor blood supply and the forces acting on the fracture fragments. In addition to the flexion deformity, the distal pole of the scaphoid is subject to a pronation moment resulting in a three-dimensional deformity.[19] Scaphoid fractures heal by primary bone healing or intramembranous ossification without the benefit of fracture callous to provide initial stability. Stability of the fracture fragments determines the amount of strain at the fracture site. The amount of strain determines the type of healing. Strain less than 2% results in primary bone healing. Strain between 2% and 10% results in secondary bone healing. Finally, with strain more than 10% bone cannot heal and fibrous or granulation tissue is formed.[20] The additional demands put on the athlete's wrist can result in a wide range of traumatic lesions in the carpus.

DIAGNOSIS AND WORKUP
History

The athlete with an injured wrist should have a thorough history and physical examination. In particular, suspicion of a carpal injury should accompany a mechanism consistent with a fall with forced hyperextension or palmar-flexion, such as a collision or a direct blow to the wrist from a ball, a stick, or another player (**Fig. 2**). Rettig has previously stated that any athlete with radial wrist pain should carry the diagnosis of scaphoid fracture until proven otherwise.[21] Although injuries are more common during competition, many injuries often occur during practice or unsupervised settings and may go unnoticed. Some patients will present with a less acute history of trauma with chronic wrist discomfort, lack of range of motion, inability to perform push-ups, or difficulty with gripping a club or racket.[21]

Physical Examination

A thorough physical examination of the wrist should always be done in the workup of wrist pain and injury in the athlete. The degree and location of swelling and passive and active range of motion should be noted. Tenderness with palpation in the anatomic snuffbox or pain with axial loading applied by the thumb is often found with scaphoid fractures. There are also specific examination tests for carpal instability. Watson's test for scapholunate instability involves the examiner placing volar pressure over the athlete's scaphoid tubercle as the wrist is brought from ulnar to radial deviation.[22] Partial tears will illicit pain over the scapholunate articulation whereas complete tears will produce an audible clunk as the scaphoid is dorsally subluxed and then reduced into the radial fossa as the volar pressure is released. In the evaluation for lunotriquetral instability, Kleinman has described the "shear" test in which the examiner stabilizes the radiolunate articulation with the forearm in neutral rotation and with the contralateral hand loads the triquetrum in the anteroposterior plane, creating shear across the lunotriquetral joint that can produce a spectrum of symptoms from pain to an audible clunk.[23] A full neurovascular examination is also important because the more severe forms of carpal instability and perilunate dislocations can be associated with acute median neuropathy.

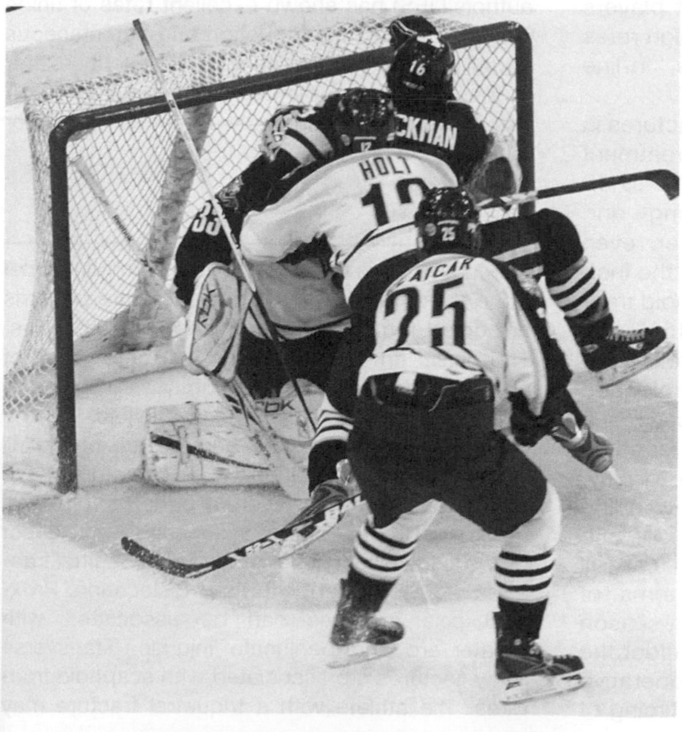

Fig. 2. Hockey, a stick sport, also involves high-energy collisions. Hand and wrist injuries can result from a direct blow from a stick, a collision with another player, or a fall on the ice. Although hyperextension injuries are more prone to produce carpal fractures or ligament injuries, stick sports such as baseball or golf or tennis can result in hook of the hamate fracture. (*Courtesy of* Steven Conn, BA and Sam Rubin, BA, New Haven, CT; with permission from Yale Athletics.)

Diagnostic Imaging

At the authors' institution, plain radiographs of the athlete's wrist include posteroanterior (PA), lateral, oblique, clenched fist, and PA with ulnar deviation views along with contralateral films to detect subtle fractures or widening indicative of ligamentous injury. MRI is more sensitive for the evaluation of both ligamentous injury and occult scaphoid fractures as compared to plain radiographs and bone scintigraphy.[24,25] CT scan may be useful in evaluating carpal fractures particularly with sagittal images parallel to the long axis of the scaphoid to help define collapse or "humpback" deformity.[26]

FRACTURES OF THE CARPUS
Scaphoid

The scaphoid is the most common carpal bone to sustain a fracture and represents 60% to 70% of all carpal fractures.[27] In athletes, scaphoid fractures have been most commonly associated with contact sports such as football, and in sports with potentially high-impact falls such as basketball, in-line skating, snowboarding, and rodeo-riding. A 1-year survey of hand injuries at the Methodist Sports Medicine Center in Indianapolis found that scaphoid fractures accounted for 19% of all fractures with the highest occurrences in basketball and football players.[28] Reister estimated the incidence of scaphoid fractures in college level American football at 1% of players per year.[29] Others have found relatively high rates of scaphoid fracture in snowboarders, in-line skating, and rodeo-riders.[30–32]

The management of acute scaphoid fractures in athletes remains a challenge. Traditional treatment of the acute scaphoid fracture involves 8 to 12 weeks or more of immobilization in long- and short-arm thumb spica casts.[33] However, even with extended periods of immobilization, the incidence of nonunion in nondisplaced scaphoid fractures has been reported to be as high as 15%, and with any fracture displacement can increase the incidence of nonunion to 50%.[34–36] Prolonged immobilization in the athletic population can result in stiffness and muscle atrophy that can lengthen the period of therapy in order to return to play. For the athlete, decreasing the risk for developing a nonunion, decreasing the time to union, and decreasing the length of immobilization can all be important issues to consider in terms of decreasing the time to return to play. In-season injury versus off-season injury can also affect the athlete's decision-making in terms of operative versus nonoperative treatment and also timing of the surgery. Therefore, options for treatment can include nonoperative treatment as definitive management, nonoperative treatment until surgery in the off-season, acute operative treatment. Nonoperative treatment with immobilization until later surgery has several factors to consider in terms of return to sport. First, immobilization of nondisplaced or minimally displaced fractures carries the risk for further displacement and possible carpal instability. Also, return to play with immobilization is sport-specific. The National Football League, the National Collegiate Athletic Association, and the National Federation of State High School Associations allow football players to compete while wearing splints made of rigid materials if the splint is covered by a half inch of cell foam.[37] Other sports have state-specific rules, and local authorities should be contacted for further details before making recommendations to patients and their families. Return-to-play guidelines are summarized in **Table 1**.

Operative treatment of acute scaphoid fractures has also evolved. Rettig and Kollias[38] showed that open reduction and internal fixation through a volar Russe approach with the Herbert technique of acute scaphoid fractures in athletes allowed them to return to sport at an average of 5.8 weeks.[33,35] Early range of motion can help to decrease adhesions and reduce stiffness. Open volar approaches are associated with disruption of the extrinsic palmar ligaments and instability has been reported after open repair.[39] One of the authors (JFS) has shown excellent rates of union with an arthroscopic reduction and percutaneous dorsal fixation.[40] This technique is described later in the article and potentially allows for less soft tissue dissection and early return to sport for athletes.

Triquetrum

The triquetrum is the second most common carpal bone to be fractured. Two main fracture patterns are dorsal rim chip fractures and body fractures. The dorsal rim chip fractures can be a result of an avulsion of the dorsal radiotriquetral ligament, compression against the ulnar styloid, or the dorsal proximal edge of the hamate striking the triquetrum in ulnar-deviation.[41] Body fractures have been divided into six different patterns.[42] Medial tuberosity fractures are associated with direct blows to the ulnar border of the wrist. Sagittal fractures are associated with axial dislocation. Proximal pole fractures can be associated with greater arc and perilunate injuries. Transverse body fractures are associated with scaphoid fractures. The athlete with a triquetral fracture may

Table 1
Guidelines for return to play after treatment of scaphoid waist fractures with a headless compression screw

Sport and Position	Timing of Return to Play After Treatment with a Headless Compression Screw for Scaphoid Waist Fractures[b]	Treatment
Football		
Line	2 weeks	Playing cast
Skilled	2–4 weeks[a]	No cast (brace—2 weeks)
Basketball	2 weeks	No cast
Baseball	2–4 weeks	No cast
Soccer	2 weeks	Playing cast
Lacrosse	2–4 weeks	Possible playing cast
Hockey	2–4 weeks	Possible playing cast
Snowboarding	4 weeks	Playing cast Wrist guard
Skiing	2–4 weeks	Playing cast
In-line skating	2–4 weeks	Playing cast Wrist guard
Weight lifting	8–12 weeks; CT[a]	No cast
Wrestling	8–12 weeks; CT[a]	No cast
Field hockey	2–4 weeks	Possible cast Wrist guard
Gymnastics	8–12 weeks; CT[a]	No cast
Rodeo	4–8 weeks; CT[a]	Playing cast Wrist guard
Boxing	6–12 weeks; CT[a]	No cast

[a] CT scan—identify 50% bridging bone.
[b] For scaphoid proximal pole fractures, add 4 weeks to timing of return to play. CT scans must be done to confirm healing prior to return to play.
From Slade JF, Magit DP, Geissler WB. Scaphoid fractures in athletes. Atlas of the Hand Clinics 2006;11:41; with permission.

show tenderness to palpation just distal to the ulnar styloid with the hand in radial deviation. Treatment generally consists of cast immobilization for 4 to 6 weeks. Body fractures with associated carpal instability or other carpal fractures may be treated with open reduction and internal fixation. Painful nonunion fragments can be excised if necessary.

Hamate

Hamate fractures are divided into two patterns: hook of the hamate and body fractures. Hook of the hamate fractures are more common in athletes. They are classically described as resulting from direct impact from a golf club handle, hockey stick, or repetitive trauma from a tennis racquet or shearing applied by the ring and small finger flexor tendons.[43] Ulnar nerve symptoms may occur with these injuries and should heighten

suspicion of these often missed injuries. Athletes with these injuries may have weakened grasp and hypothenar pain. Resisted little finger flexion and axial loading of the fourth or fifth metacarpal should be tested. These fractures are often missed on conventional radiographic views. A carpal tunnel or supinated oblique view should be done with CT scan providing the most definitive radiographic evidence. Athletes with hook of the hamate fractures can be treated with cast immobilization, closed reduction and pinning, open reduction and internal fixation (ORIF), and late excision of symptomatic nonunions. Hirano and Inoue found in their series that associated neurovascular and musculotendinous injuries were most predictive of less favorable functional results.[44] Many authors recommend excision with return to sport in 7 to 10 weeks.[43,45] Excision or ORIF may be complicated by decreased grip strength secondary to the removal of the attachment for the transverse carpal ligament, pisohamate ligament, and flexor and opponens digiti minimi muscles.

Lunate

Isolated fracture of the lunate in athletes is rare. Repetitive or previous trauma may put athletes at risk for avascular necrosis of the lunate or Kienböck disease. Some authors feel that athletes requiring extreme weight bearing with the wrist in extension, as with gymnastics and weight lifting, are at increased risk for this disease.[46] Athletes with tenderness at their lunate should be fully evaluated for possible carpal instability or perilunate dislocation. Radiographs may be negative in patients with early Kienböck disease. MRI is needed for definitive diagnosis. The treatment of avascular necrosis of the lunate depends on the stage and varies from carpal or radial shortening procedures in early stages without significant degenerative changes to salvage procedures for pain control without significant promise of return to previous level of range of motion, strength, or return to sporting level.[1,47]

Capitate

Capitate fractures in isolation are also rare and usually occur in association with perilunate dislocations and carpal instability. One unique pattern is the scaphocapitate syndrome which involves a trans-scaphoid, trans-capitate, perilunate fracture dislocation pattern often with the proximal fragment of the transverse capitate fracture rotated 180 degrees.[48] These result from a fall on an extended and radially deviated wrist. The capitate fracture may need open reduction and internal fixation or percutaneous fixation in association with surgical treatment of the associated perilunate dislocation and scaphoid fracture.

Pisiform

The pisiform is a sesamoid in the flexor carpi ulnaris tendon that when fractured can disrupt this tendon. Transverse fractures can result from direct trauma or by extreme flexor carpi ulnaris contraction. These injuries are associated with racquet sport athletes.[49] Athletes may have ulnar-sided wrist pain, weak grip strength, or decreased range of motion. These fractures may be missed on conventional radiographs, so CT scan or MRI may be needed for diagnosis. Pisotriquetral chondromalacia, tendon subluxation, or osteoarthritis may develop if a malunion or nonunion develops. Acute injuries may be treated with immobilization for 4 to 6 weeks. Chronic symptomatic injuries can be treated with pisiform excision.[50]

CARPAL LIGAMENT INJURY AND INSTABILITY
Scapholunate Ligament

Scapholunate dissociation is the most common form of carpal instability in athletes and usually results from excessive wrist extension with the wrist in ulnar deviation.[8,18,51] A spectrum of injury exists from sprain to partial tear to complete tear with or without other associated carpal ligament and instability patterns. Chronic and complete injuries will result in progressive flexion of the scaphoid, extension of the lunotriquetral complex, and dorsal intercalated segment instability.[8] Athletes with these injuries may give a history with the fall mechanism as previously mentioned in the acute setting or past history. Physical examination findings may include pain dorsally over the scapholunate interval, decreased grip strength, or decreased range of motion. These injuries may be misdiagnosed as subacute wrist sprains by coaches, trainers, and physicians alike. The Watson shift test described previously may be positive for pain or audible clunk. Standard radiographs should be done in addition to a PA view with clenched fist to assess for static and dynamic scapholunate diastasis and should be compared to the contralateral side. MRI is more sensitive and specific to accurately distinguish these injuries from other carpal ligament and tendon injuries.

Arthroscopy is considered the gold standard to assess for dynamic instability (**Fig. 3**). Geissler and colleagues have defined an arthroscopic instability classification.[52] Grade I is defined as attenuation or hemorrhage of the ligament visualized from the radiocarpal side. Grade II adds incongruency with a gap less than the width of a probe between the carpal bones. Grade III has incongruency seen from both the midcarpal and radiocarpal sides, and a probe can be passed through the intercarpal space (**Fig. 4**). Grade IV has gross instability with manipulation, and the arthroscope can be passed through the intercarpal space. Operative treatments can vary from dorsal capsulodesis, such as the Blatt or Mayo procedures, to tenodesis, such as the Brunelli procedure, where a strip of the flexor carpi radialis is brought volarly through a tunnel in the scaphoid and then dorsally to attach to the distal radius or the lunate to limit scaphoid flexion.[53–55] Newer techniques involve reconstruction of the ligament with bone-retinaculum-bone autografts.[56,57] Chronic scapholunate instability and resulting DISI deformity can lead to arthritic changes in which salvage procedures such as partial wrist arthrodesis or proximal row carpectomy may become the only option for pain control. The key

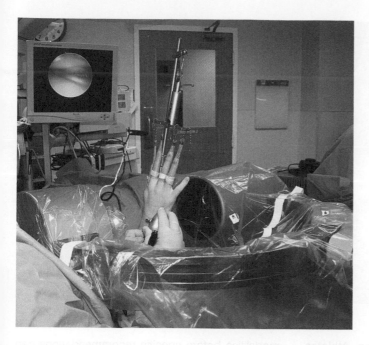

Fig. 3. Arthroscopy is the gold standard to assess for carpal ligament injuries. Geissler and colleagues have defined an arthroscopic instability classification. (*From* Geissler WB, Freeland AE, Savoie FH, et al. Intracarpal soft-tissue lesions associated with an intra-articular fracture of the distal end of the radius. J Bone Joint Surg Am 1996;78:357–65.)

to treating the athlete with this injury is early diagnosis and treatment.

Lunotriquetral Ligament

Lunotriquetral instability is the second most common form of carpal instability but is approximately six times less common than scapholunate instability.[58] The mechanism of injury is similar, with the athlete usually suffering a fall with wrist extension and radial deviation with intercarpal pronation instead of supination. Athletes will describe ulnar-sided wrist pain, grip weakness, and possible clicking. The Watson shift test and Kleinman shear test may help distinguish scapholunate from lunotriquetral injury. Radiographic examinations are notoriously unreliable to detect these injuries accurately, and even MRI may be unreliable. Luckily, lunotriquetral injuries are less likely to develop degenerative changes and immobilization can lead to acceptable outcomes in 80% of patients.[1,59] Arthroscopic evaluation is an excellent modality for diagnosis, and debridement of partial tears has shown good results.[60] Athletes can usually expect to return to sport approximately 6 to 8 weeks after arthroscopic debridement.[1] Those who fail initial management with arthroscopic treatment may benefit from ulnar shortening osteotomy which reduces forces on the ulnar side of the carpus and increases stability by tensioning the ulnar sided ligaments.[61] However, an athlete can expect a longer recovery time of 3 to 6 months for this treatment modality before returning to sport.[1]

Perilunate Dislocations

Perilunate dislocations represent the most severe of carpal ligament injuries (**Fig. 5**). Mayfield had originally described a reproducible pattern of injuries starting with scapholunate diastasis or scaphoid fracture, proceeding to capitate fracture or ligament injury, then lunotriquetral ligament failure or triquetrum fracture, and finally in the most severe injuries complete dislocation of the lunate into the carpal tunnel.[17] Once again, the mechanism of injury is extreme wrist extension

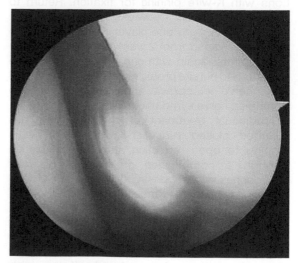

Fig. 4. Arthroscopic examination from the radial midcarpal joint diagnosis, a grade IIItear of the SLIO ligament.

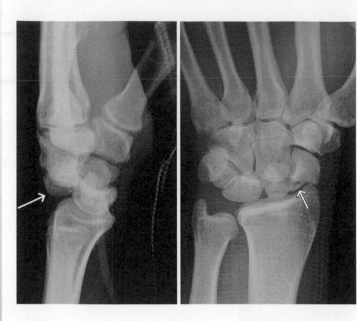

Fig. 5. Perilunate dislocations represent the most severe of carpal ligament injuries. The most common of the trans-scaphoid perilunate dislocation is the dorsal translocation. The arc of injury travels through the scaphoid, fracturing its waist, and commonly exits through the lunotriquetral interosseous (LTIO) ligament, resulting in a tear of this ligament.

in ulnar deviation with carpal supination. Athletes with these injuries usually describe a high force axial loading moment on their extended wrist. They will have significant swelling and discomfort and they must be evaluated for median and ulnar neuropathy, which may necessitate emergent decompression. All perilunate dislocations require immediate closed reduction as soon as possible with emergent open reduction for those whose closed reduction attempts are unsuccessful.

A 5-year retrospective review of National Football League team physicians found 10 of these injuries from 1986 to 1990.[62] These were treated with a variety of closed and open operative reductions with K-wire pinning for fixation. Return to practice varied from 1.5 weeks to the next season for 4 patients, with one player retiring. Return to game play varied from 2 weeks to next season in two patients, again with one player retiring. Two patients had pin site problems, one had a superficial radial nerve neurapraxia, and one patient went on to median nerve sympathetic dystrophy.

Traditional treatment of these injuries has included closed reduction with percutaneous pinning to open reduction and internal fixation through a combination of dorsal and volar approaches with reconstruction or repair of ligamentous injuries.[63] Arthroscopically aided closed reduction and percutaneous pinning or screw fixation with limited exposures for ligament repair have been described and offer the athlete newer treatment options that may aid in minimizing soft tissue dissection and adhesions and could offer a quicker return to sport (**Fig. 6**).[64,65] Further studies will need to evaluate the long-term results of these treatment modalities before specific recommendations can be made for athletes in terms of return to play.

WRIST INJURY PREVENTION

With so much attention focused on diagnosis and treatment of wrist injuries, one must also examine potential preventive measures. There is controversy in the literature as to whether bracing or wrist guards are effective in preventing wrist injuries. One cadaveric model showed decreased carpal fractures, ligament injuries, and capsular tears with wrist bracing.[66] However, others have not shown significant differences in preventing wrist fractures with in-line skating type wrist guards.[67] Prospective and retrospective studies in European snowboarders have show that wrist guards significantly decrease the incidence of wrist fractures and injuries.[68,69] There is some concern that wrist guards may just change the area of force transmission from a fall. They may produce a stress riser at their proximal edge, and one study reported open forearm fractures as a result of in-line skaters' using wrist guards.[70] New wrist guards may be tailored for an athlete's specific demands and potential for injury in the hope that they can decrease carpal injuries but not diminish an athlete's mobility and ability to perform.

DIAGNOSTIC WRIST ARTHROSCOPY AND PERCUTANEOUS REDUCTION AND FIXATION TECHNIQUES

Diagnostic wrist arthroscopy has become an important part of the surgical evaluation of carpal

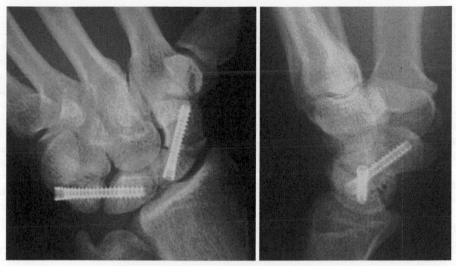

Fig. 6. Dorsal trans-scaphoid perilunate dislocation treated with arthroscopically aided closed reduction and percutaneous screw fixation with limited exposures for the LTIO ligament repair using Mitek anchors. The LTIO ligament repair is protected for 6 months with a headless screw, which will be removed later. This offers the athlete newer treatment options that may aid in minimizing soft tissue dissection and adhesions and could offer a quicker return to sport. (*Left panel from* Weil WM, Slade JF, Trumble TE. Open and arthroscopic treatment of perilunate injuries. Clin Orthop Relat Res 2006;445:120–32; *right panel from* Park MJ, Ahn JH. Arthroscopically assisted reduction and percutaneous fixation of dorsal perilunate dislocations and fracture-dislocations. Arthroscopy 2005;21(9):1153.)

injuries and an adjuvant for the confirmation of fracture and ligamentous reductions (**Fig. 7**). Although open techniques have the advantage of direct visualization and the ability to address several related carpal injuries through one exposure, arthroscopically assisted percutaneous and minimally invasive techniques have the potential advantage of less soft-tissue dissection, which could lead to decreased postoperative immobilization and less resultant stiffness and atrophy. These potential advantages are intriguing for all patients but especially for the athlete. Prolonged immobilization, larger casts that interfere with return to sport, and lengthy rehabilitation protocols can all delay a return to preinjury performance. The authors present a set of techniques for

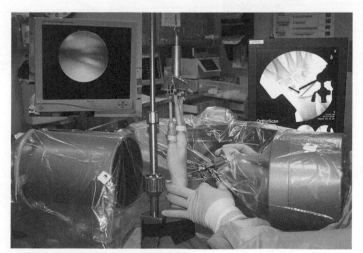

Fig. 7. Small joint arthroscopy is used in conjunction with mini-fluoroscopy to surgically evaluate the wrist for carpal injuries. The positioning of the imaging unit perpendicular to the carpus provides for accurate evaluation of injuries and confirmation of reduction and implant placement.

arthroscopic evaluation of carpal injuries along with percutaneous reduction and fixation techniques for scaphoid fractures and associated carpal fractures and ligament tears.[2]

Imaging

Once the patient has been placed on the standard operative table, with a hand table extension on the operative side and with a tourniquet placed on the upper arm prior to prepping, then an examination under anesthesia is done to check for possible ligamentous instability as compared to the presumed normal contralateral wrist. The hand is then placed in the wrist traction tower if diagnostic arthroscopy is to be done first. A mini-fluoroscopy receiver is brought in a sterile cover and placed horizontally or parallel with the floor. A fluoroscopic survey of the carpus is then performed and correlated with findings from preoperative examinations, imaging, and examination under anesthesia.

Special attention is paid to fracture location and displacement especially with dynamic stress. Dynamic instability patterns can also be evaluated and defined at this time. If a scaphoid fracture is present, then the central axis of the scaphoid must be found as the next step. The wrist should be pronated and flexed until the reduced scaphoid appears as a "ring," with the direction of fluoroscopy now representing both the central axis of the scaphoid and the proper direction for screw placement.

Dorsal Guidewire Placement for Scaphoid Fixation

With the central axis now defined by the fluoroscopy, a 0.045" K-wire is placed from a dorsal position volarly and radially along the long axis of the scaphoid (**Fig. 8**). The wrist must be adequately held in a flexed position to avoid bending or breaking the guidewire. The guidewire is then advanced through the trapezium and the skin at the radial aspect near the carpometacarpal joint. The wire is advanced in the volar direction until the trailing end of the wire clears the radiocarpal joint and the wrist is permitted to return to full extension. Central alignment of the guide pin can now be confirmed in multiple fluoroscopic planes.

Percutaneous Carpal Fracture Reduction

If a displaced scaphoid is present, then the next necessary step should be a closed reduction using a percutaneous technique. The guidewire should be advanced volarly and radially into the distal segment of scaphoid fracture. Under fluoroscopic guidance, percutaneous dorsal 0.062" K-wires are placed in the scaphoid fragments as "joysticks" to allow for closed reduction. Often the distal segment needs to be extended and the proximal fragment flexed. The previously placed central guidewire is then advanced in the reverse direction dorsally to cross the now reduced scaphoid fracture. A second parallel guidewire is often needed to hold these unstable displaced fractures.

This technique can be repeated if other displaced fractures in the carpus are noted. Smaller

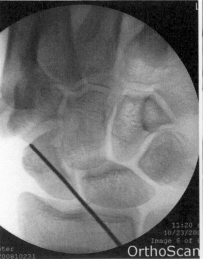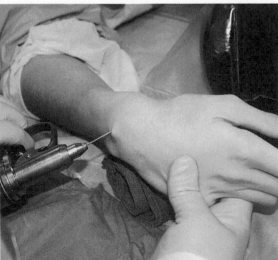

Fig. 8. Guidewire placement for scaphoid fixation: The central axis is defined by fluoroscopy, a 0.045" K-wire is placed from a dorsal position volarly and radially along the long axis of the scaphoid. The wrist must be flexed to avoid bending or breaking the guidewire.

K-wires may be more appropriate for the lunate reduction maneuvers. The lead author (JFS) often uses small cannulated compression screws to hold the reduction of other carpal fractures and also for the reduction of ligament injuries such as lunotriquetral instability. Many other authors advocate the use of percutaneous K-wire fixation. In either technique, K-wires are placed initially with the screw fixation technique utilizing arthroscopically aided confirmation of reduction before final screw placement.

A limited dorsal incision can be made dorsally directly over the torn or unstable ligament after preliminary fixation to allow for direct repair with suture anchor fixation or augmentation with autograft or allograft.

Arthroscopic Evaluation

Arthroscopic evaluation can be done either initially, before any fracture reduction or fixation is attempted, or after provisional fixation of the scaphoid fracture.[71] The midcarpal and radiocarpal portals are located under fluoroscopic guidance with 19-gauge needles. The small joint arthroscope is placed in the mid-carpal and radiocarpal portals to confirm fracture reduction. The integrity of the scapholunate and lunotriquetral interossei ligaments, along with the triangular fibrocartilage complex, and cartilaginous surfaces of

intra-articular carpal bones, can be evaluated. A small snap forceps can be inserted through these portals to dynamically assess the integrity of the ligament complexes which can be confirmed fluoroscopically. The 3, 4 and 4, 5 and the 6R portals are also utilized to assess the radiocarpal joint. Once final reduction positions have been confirmed and all intra-articular pathology that can be addressed through the arthroscope has been achieved, attention is turned to final screw fixation.

Screw Fixation

Scaphoid or other carpal screw length can be measured by first ensuring that the guidewire is placed adjacent to the distal cortex. A second wire is placed parallel and up to the proximal pole of the scaphoid and the difference is measured. A screw should be selected that allows 2 mm of clearance both proximally and distally. Implantation of a screw that is too long is the most common complication of percutaneous screw fixation. A cannulated drill is then advanced by hand and is confirmed by fluoroscopic imaging (**Fig. 9**). The screw is then inserted either dorsally or volarly. Dorsal implantation is favored for proximal pole fractures and volar implantation for distal pole scaphoid fractures. Other carpal bone screw implantation will depend on carpal bone and

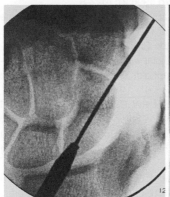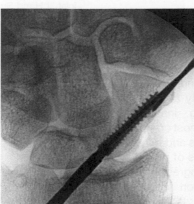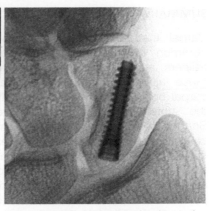

Fig. 9. After placement of a central axis guidewire. Two wires, of equal length, are placed. The first leading edge stops at the distal scaphoid; the second leading edge is placed at the proximal pole. The difference between the two wires is the scaphoid length. A headless cannulated compression screw, 4 mm shorter, is selected for implantation. A small incision is made at the base of the central axis guidewire. Blunt dissection is made to the wrist capsule, ensuring no tendons have been impaled. If a tendon has been skewed, the wire is withdrawn and the tendon retracted. A reamer is used to breach the proximal pole, and a headless cannulated screw is implanted. One caveat to be considered when repairing the young is that young bone has higher density, which may result in "push-off" when implanting a screw. To prevent fracture separation, a 0.062" K-wire joystick is inserted into the distal fracture fragment to apply a counter-force as the screw is inserted. A standard size headless compression screw is used because it is stronger than a mini-screw and better resists micro-motion at the fracture site. The screw is implanted using imaging to ensure that the screw is not overdriven into the scaphotrapezial joint. Once the screw is implanted, its position is checked using imaging, with the guidewire advanced volarly so the wrist can be extended.

fracture configuration. Once all fractures have been addressed with screw fixation and reduction and hardware placement is satisfactorily assessed arthroscopically, the guidewires are removed.

POSTOPERATIVE CARE AND RETURN TO PLAY

The postoperative treatment after a carpal fracture, fractures, or ligament injury treated by arthroscopically assisted percutaneous reduction is dictated by the soft-tissue injury that is present. An isolated scaphoid waist fracture without ligament injury can be started on an immediate range of motion protocol with proximal pole fractures immobilized for 1 month postoperatively.[2] If there has been significant ligament injury, especially injury necessitating surgical reduction and fixation, the athlete needs to be immobilized for 6 weeks postoperatively followed by a protected motion program. A strengthening program is begun for scaphoid fracture to assist with axial loading to stimulate healing. However, contact sports and heavy lifting should be restricted until CT scans confirm healing by bridging callous. The lead author (JFS) has previously developed algorithms for return to sport for specific sports along with their specific restrictions on types of immobilization.[2] These are summarized in **Table 1**.

SUMMARY

Carpal fractures and ligamentous injuries are common in athletes and require physicians, trainers, and therapists who treat and diagnosis these injuries to have an understanding of the carpal bone anatomy and vascularity along with the potential for progression to instability. Scaphoid fractures are certainly the most common carpal bone to be fractured in athletes and may be the most challenging to treat in terms of potential for malunion, nonunion, and progression to arthritic collapse. However, attention must be paid to other potential carpal fractures and ligaments in the injured athlete's wrist. An athlete's immediate health and safety along with seasonal and career goals must be considered by the treating physician and surgeon in deciding on treatment options that can range from nonoperative immobilization with casting and bracing to operative treatment with classic open exposures and newer arthroscopically assisted techniques, which were described in detail. Research is still needed to further investigate the optimal treatments of all carpal injuries in athletes along with designing new means to prevent these injuries.

REFERENCES

1. Rettig AC. Athletic injuries of the wrist and hand. Part I: traumatic injuries of the wrist. Am J Sports Med 2003;31(6):1038–48.
2. Slade JF, Magit DP, Geissler WB. Scaphoid fractures in athletes. Atlas of the Hand Clinics 2006; 11:27–44.
3. Buterbaugh GA, Brown TR, Horn PC. Ulnar-sided wrist pain in athletes. Clin Sports Med 1998;17: 567–83.
4. Brophy RH, Lyman S, Chehab EL, et al. Predictive value of prior injury on career in professional American football is affected by player position. Am J Sports Med 2009;37(4):768–75.
5. Taleisnik J. The ligaments of the wrist. J Hand Surg 1976;1:1612–32.
6. Berger RA, Landsmeer JM. The palmar radiocarpal ligaments: a study of adult and fetal human wrist joints. J Hand Surg 1990;15:847–54.
7. Bednar JM, Osterman AL. Carpal instability: evaluation and treatment. J Am Acad Orthop Surg 1993; 1(1):10–7.
8. Linscheid RL, Dobyns JH, Beabout JW, et al. Traumatic instability of the wrist: diagnosis, classification, and patho mechanics. J Bone Joint Surg Am 1972; 54:1612–32.
9. Gelberman RH, Menon J. The vascularity of the scaphoid bone. J Hand Surg 1980;5(5):508–13.
10. Ritt MJ, Berger RA, Kauer JM. The gross and histologic anatomy of the ligaments of the capitohamate joint. J Hand Surg 1996;21:1022–8.
11. Berger RA. The anatond basic biomechanics of the wrist joint. J Hand Ther 1996;9:84–93.
12. Gilford WW, Bolton RH, Lambrinudi C. The mechanism of the wrist joint with special reference to fractures of the scaphoid. Guys Hosp Rep 1943;92: 52–9.
13. Palmer AK, Werner RW. Biomechanics of the distal radioulnar joint. Clin Orthop 1984;187:26–35.
14. Viegas SF, Patterson R, Todd PD, et al. Load mechanics of the midcarpal joint. J Hand Surg 1993;18:14–28.
15. Weber ER, Chao EY. An experimental approach to the mechanism of scaphoid waist fractures. J Hand Surg 1978;3(2):142–8.
16. Slade JF, Jaskwhich D. Percutaneous fixation of scaphoid fractures. Hand Clin 2001;17(4):553–74.
17. Mayfield JK. Mechanism of carpal injuries. Clin Orthop 1980;149:45–54.
18. Mayfield JK, Johnson RP, Kilcoyne RK. Carpal dislocations: pathomechanics and progressive perilunar instability. J Hand Surg 1980;5:226–41.
19. Belsole RJ, Hilbelink DR, Llewellyn JA, et al. Computed analyses of the pathomechanics of scaphoid waist nonunions. J Hand Surg 1991; 16(5):899–906.

20. Egol KA, Kubiak EN, Fulkerson E, et al. Biomechanics of locked plates and screws. J Orthop Trauma 2004;18(8):488–93.

21. Rettig AC. Management of acute scaphoid fractures. Hand Clin 2000;16(3):381–95.

22. Watson HK, Ashmead DT, Makhlouf MV. Examination of the scaphoid. J Hand Surg 1988;13:657–60.

23. Schmidt CC, Kleinman WB. Lunatotriquetral fusion. Atlas Hand Clin 1998;3:115–27.

24. Hunter JC, Escobedo EM, Wilson AJ, et al. MR imaging of clinically suspected scaphoid fractures. Am J Roentgenol 1997;168(5):1287–93.

25. Fowler C, Sullivan B, Williams LA, et al. A comparison of bone scintigraphy and MRI in the early diagnosis of the occult scaphoid waist fracture. Skeletal Radiol 1998;27:683–7.

26. Sanders WE. Evaluation of the humpback scaphoid by computed tomography in the longitudinal axial plane of the scaphoid. J Hand Surg 1988;13:182–7.

27. Borgeskov S, Christiansen B, Kjaer A, et al. Fractures of the carpal bones. Acta Orthop Scand 1966;37(3):276–87.

28. Strickland JW, Rettig AC. Hand injuries in athletes. Philadelphia: WB Saunders Co.; 1992. p. 37–48.

29. Reister JN, Baker BE, Mosher JF, et al. A review of scaphoid fracture healing in competitive athletes. Am J Sports Med 1985;13(3):159–61.

30. Nguyen D, Letts M. In-line skating injuries in children: a 10-year review. J Pediatr Orthop 2001; 21(5):613–8.

31. Sasaki K, Takagi M, Kiyoshige Y, et al. Snowboarder's wrist: its severity compared with Alpine skiing. J Trauma 1999;46(6):1059–61.

32. Meyers MC, Sterling JC, Souryal TO. Radiographic findings of the upper extremity in collegiate rodeo athletes. Med Sci Sports Exerc 2003;35(4):543–7.

33. Russe O. Fractures of the carpal navicular diagnosis, non-operative treatment, and operative treatment. J Bone Joint Surg Am 1960;42:759–68.

34. Kuschner S, Lane CS, Brien WW, et al. Scaphoid fractures and scaphoid nonunion. Diagnosis and treatment. Orthop Rev 1994;23(11):861–71.

35. Herbert T, Fisher W. Management of the fractured scaphoid using a new bone screw. J Bone Joint Surg Br 1984;66:114–23.

36. Herbert T. Use of the Herbert bone screw in surgery of the wrist. Clin Orthop Relat Res 1986; 202:79–92.

37. Alexy C, DeCarlo M. Rehabilitation and use of protective devices in hand and wrist injuries. Clin Sports Med 1998;17(3):635–55.

38. Rettig AC, Kollias SC. Internal fixation of acute stable scaphoid fractures in the athlete. Am J Sports Med 1996;24(2):182–6.

39. Filan SL, Herbert TJ. Herbert screw fixation of scaphoid fractures. J Bone Joint Surg Br 1996; 78(4):519–29.

40. Slade JF, Gillon T. Retrospective review of 234 scaphoid fractures and nonunions treated with arthroscopy for union and complications. Scand J Surg 2008;97(4):280–9.

41. Hocker K, Menschik A. Chip fractures of the triquetrum. Mechanism, classification and results. J Hand Surg Br 1994;19(5):584–8.

42. Garcias-Elias M. Carpal bone fractures (excluding the scaphoid). In: Watson HK, Weinzweig J, editors. The wrist. Philadelphia: Lippincott Williams & Wilkins; 2001. p. 173–86.

43. Stark HH, Jobe FW, Boyes JH, et al. Fracture of the hook of the hamate in athletes. J Bone Joint Surg Am 1977;59:575–82.

44. Hirano K, Inoue G. Classification and treatment of hamate fractures. Hand Surg 2005;10(2–3):151–7.

45. Parker RD, Berkowitz MS, Brahms MA, et al. Hook of the hamate fractures in athletes. Am J Sports Med 1986;14:517–23.

46. Burger H, Muller EJ, Kalicke T. Avascular necrosis of the capitate in athletes. Sportverletz Sportschaden 2006;20(2):91–5.

47. Allan CH, Joshi A, Lichtman DM. Kienböck's disease: diagnosis and treatment. J Am Acad Orthop Surg 2001;9:128–36.

48. Resnik CS, Gelberman RH, Resnick D. Transscaphoid, transcapitate, perilunate fracture dislocation (scaphocapitate syndrome). Skeletal Radiol 1983; 9(3):192–4.

49. Helal B. Racquet player's pisiform. Hand 1978;10: 87–90.

50. Palmieri TJ. Pisiform area pain treatment by pisiform excision. J Hand Surg 1982;7A:477–80.

51. Lewis DM, Osterman AL. Scapholunate instability in athletes. Clin Sports Med 2001;20(1):131–40.

52. Geissler WB, Freeland AE, Savoie FH, et al. Intracarpal soft-tissue lesions associated with an intra-articular fracture of the distal end of the radius. J Bone Joint Surg Am 1996;78:357–65.

53. Blatt G. Capsulodesis in reconstructive hand surgery. Dorsal capsulodesis for the unstable scaphoid and volar capsulodesis following excision of the distal ulna. Hand Clin 1987;3:81–102.

54. Walsh JJ, Berger RA, Cooney WP. Current status of scapholunate interosseous ligament injuries. J Am Acad Orthop Surg 2002;10:32–42.

55. Brunelli GA, Brunelli GR. A new technique to correct carpal instability with scaphoid rotary subluxation: a preliminary report. J Hand Surg Am 1995;20: S82–5.

56. Weiss AP. Scapholunate ligament reconstruction using a bone-retinaculum-bone autograft. J Hand Surg 1998;23:205–15.

57. Wolf JM, Weiss AP. Bone-retinaculum-bone reconstruction of scapholunate ligament injuries. Orthop Clin North Am 2001;32:241–6.

58. Trumble TE, Bour CJ, Smith RJ, et al. Kinematics of the ulnar carpus related to the volar intercalated segment instability pattern. J Hand Surg Am 1990; 15:384–92.

59. Cohen MS. Ligamentous injuries of the wrist in the athlete. Clin Sports Med 1998;17:533–52.

60. Ruch DS, Poehling GC. Arthroscopic management of partial scapholunate and lunotriquetral injuries of the wrist. J Hand Surg Am 1996;21:412–7.

61. Linscheid RL. Ulnar lengthening and shortening. Hand Clin 1987;3:69–79.

62. Raab DJ, Fischer DA, Quick DC. Lunate and perilunate dislocations in professional football players. Am J Sports Med 1994;22(6):841–5.

63. Kozin SH. Perilunate injuries. Diagnosis and treatment. J Am Acad Orthop Surg 1998;6(2):114–20.

64. Weil WM, Slade JF, Trumble TE. Open and arthroscopic treatment of perilunate injuries. Clin Orthop Relat Res 2006;445:120–32.

65. Park MJ, Ahn JH. Arthroscopically assisted reduction and percutaneous fixation of dorsal perilunate dislocations and fracture-dislocations. Arthroscopy 2005;21(9):1153 e1–e9.

66. Moore MS, Popovic NA, Daniel JN, et al. The effect of a wrist brace on injury patterns in experimentally produced distal radial fractures in a cadaveric model. Am J Sports Med 1997;25(3):394–401.

67. Giacobetti FB, Sharkey PF, Bos-Giacobetti MA, et al. Biomechanical analysis of the effectiveness of in-line skating wrist guards for preventing wrist fractures. Am J Sports Med 1997;25(2):223–5.

68. Machold W, Kwasny O, Gassler P, et al. Risk of injury through snowboarding. J Trauma 2000;48(6):1109–14.

69. Machold W, Kwasny O, Eisenhardt P, et al. Reduction of severe wrist injuries in snowboarding by an optimized wrist protection device: a prospective randomized trial. J Trauma 2002;52(3):517–20.

70. Cheng SL, Rajaratnam K, Raskin KB. Splint-top fracture of the forearm: a description of an in-line skating injury associated with the use of protective wrist splints. J Trauma 1995;39(6):1194–7.

71. Slade JF, Grauer JN, Mahoney JD. Arthroscopic reduction and percutaneous fixation of scaphoid fractures with a novel dorsal technique. Orthop Clin North Am 2001;32(2):247–61.

Operative Fixation of Metacarpal and Phalangeal Fractures in Athletes

William B. Geissler, MD[a,b,*]

KEYWORDS

- Hand fractures • Metacarpal fractures
- Phalangeal fractures

Metacarpal and phalangeal fractures are the most common injuries in the upper extremity.[1–3] Emmett and Breck noted that fractures of the metacarpal and phalanges accounted for approximately 10% of nearly 11,000 upper extremity fractures.[4] Metacarpal and phalangeal fractures usually occur between the ages of 10 and 40 years, are more common in men, and are a common injury in athletes.[5]

Fractures of the metacarpal and phalanges have significant economic consequences for the worker and the athlete. In 1997, Kelsey and colleagues[2] reported there were more than 17.6 million upper extremity injuries resulting in 32.5 million days of restricted activity and more than 90.5 million days off work. The cost of the injuries was approximately 18.5 million dollars.[2] Chung and Spilson estimated there were approximately 1.5 million hand and forearm fractures and that more than 600,000 of these were metacarpal and phalangeal fractures in 1998.[6]

Stable anatomic fracture restoration and early functional recovery are the goals of internal fixation of hand fractures. Open reduction and internal fixation of hand fractures has become more popular over the past 3 decades secondary to improved implant materials and designs, surgical technique, radiographic availability, and the demand for anatomic fracture restoration by the general public and athletes.[7–9] However, open reduction and internal fixation of hand fractures presents a new challenge to a hand surgeon because of the difficulty in management of small fracture fragments without devascularization. Open reduction without stable fixation increases the risk of tendon or joint adhesions adjacent to the fracture. Percutaneous techniques may offer the advantage of stable fracture fixation and early digital rehabilitation while minimizing the risks of fragment devascularization and postoperative fibroplasia.

Metacarpal and phalangeal fractures are common athletic injuries that can significantly affect the athlete's career when they occur during the season and affect the athlete's training when they occur in the off season. This situation is particularly relevant if there are complications or if fixation is not stable enough to permit early range of motion and rehabilitation. This article discusses percutaneous and open reduction techniques of hand fractures as these injuries pertain to athletes. The goal is stable fixation to allow early return to competition and rehabilitation.

UNICONDYLAR FRACTURES

London initially classified phalangeal condylar fractures in 1971.[10] Type I fractures were stable

a Section of Arthroscopic Surgery and Sports Medicine, Department of Orthopaedic Surgery and Rehabilitation, University of Mississippi Medical Center, 2500 North State Street, Jackson, MS 39216, USA
b Division of Hand and Upper Extremity Surgery, University of Mississippi Medical Center, Jackson, Mississippi
* Corresponding author. Section of Arthroscopic Surgery and Sports Medicine, Department of Orthopaedic Surgery and Rehabilitation, University of Mississippi Medical Center, 2500 North State Street, Jackson, MS 39216.
E-mail address: 3doghill@msn.com

Hand Clin 25 (2009) 409–421
doi:10.1016/j.hcl.2009.05.005
0749-0712/09/$ – see front matter © 2009 Published by Elsevier Inc.

and nondisplaced. Type II fractures were considered unstable. Type III fractures were comminuted or bicondylar. London noted that bicondylar fractures were common athletic injuries. Stark noted that unicondylar fractures of the proximal phalanx were common athletic injuries and often were missed because the athlete can often bend the finger after the initial injury.[11] Athletes frequently have a history of a finger dislocation reduced by a trainer and present to the clinic in a semi-acute state if they continue to experience pain and deformity as the fracture starts to displace.

Weiss and Hastings describe their results in a series of 38 consecutive patients who had unicondylar fractures of the proximal phalanx.[12] Nineteen patients involved in the study sustained a fracture from a ball sport. The investigators noted that unicondylar fractures tended to be more common after sports injuries when the ball came between two slightly flexed outstretched digits with high velocity, which spread the digits resulting in an oblique volar Type I fracture pattern caused by tension and rotation transmitted through the collateral ligament to the condyle involved. They described that the avulsed condyle tends to be on the outermost fingers of the hand and that the condylar toward the midline of the hand is the one that is most frequently fractured. Weiss and Hastings noted that, in their series, in those cases in which the condyle away from the midline was fractured, either a compression mechanism with the finger giving away from the midline or a tension mechanism with the finger deviating toward the midline was most likely involved. McCue and colleagues[13] concurred with those findings by Weiss and Hastings in their study of phalangeal fractures.

Unicondylar fractures of the phalanges are inherently unstable. Weiss and Hastings reported that 5 of 7 nondisplaced condylar fractures of the phalanges that were managed nonoperatively displaced during treatment. They noted that nonoperative treatment of these fractures requires extremely close follow-up due to the high likelihood of displacement.

A single Kirschner wire does not provide adequate stability of unicondylar fractures of the proximal phalanx. At least two Kirschner wires are needed for reliable fixation if this mode of stabilization is selected. Kirschner wires splint but do not compress the fracture site compared with screw fixation. Conversely, mini screws provide compression at the fracture site and a single screw centered in the condylar fragment may impart sufficient stability. Kirschner wires and mini screws may be used in combination, and two mini screws may be inserted into larger fragments. Stable fixation

seems to correlate with recovery of motion at the proximal interphalangeal (PIP) joint. However, full recovery of the PIP joint motion is an exception rather than the rule following condylar fractures, usually because of some residual extension lag or flexion contracture.

Recently, Geissler introduced the technique of headless cannulated mini screw fixation as an excellent option for intraarticular unicondylar and selected bicondylar fractures of the proximal phalanx.[14] Headless mini screws fit entirely within the bone fragment minimizing collateral ligament obstruction and irritation compared with mini screws with conventional heads. In addition, percutaneous insertion minimizes soft tissue dissection and scarring compared with a mini open procedure. Motion-restricting joint and tendon adhesions are less likely to occur. Insertion of cannulated screws allows for precise placement and simplifies the procedure significantly.

SURGICAL TECHNIQUE

Condylar fractures can usually be manually reduced within 7 to 10 days following injury (**Fig. 1**). Manipulative reduction is performed under fluoroscopic control. A dental pick, Kirschner wire, or hypodermic needle may be useful to assist reduction when closed manipulation fails to anatomically reduce the articular surface. A pointed reduction clamp or specialized fracture reduction jig may be applied to provide provisional fixation (**Fig. 2**). Adequate reduction of the condylar fracture is confirmed under fluoroscopic control both by posteroanterior (PA) and lateral radiographs. The condyle should align concentrically on lateral radiographs. A displaced condylar fracture displays a double convexity (Tushie sign) as viewed laterally if it is not fully reduced.

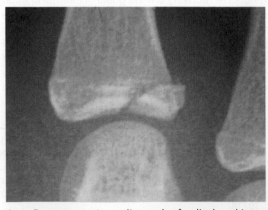

Fig. 1. Posteroanterior radiograph of a displaced intraarticular fracture of the base of the proximal phalanx to the index finger.

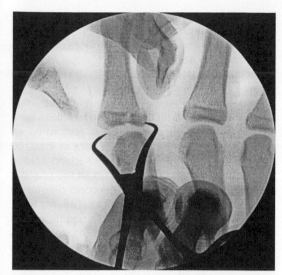

Fig. 2. Under fluoroscopy, with the aid of a towel clip, a displaced intraarticular fragment is percutaneously reduced and stabilized.

Two Kirschner wires are inserted. One guide wire is placed centrally into the condylar fragment parallel to the articular surface just distal to the origin of the collateral ligament (**Fig. 3**). This guide wire will be used for insertion of the screw. The central guide wire is advanced through the skin on the opposite side of the digit so that if the guide wire breaks during insertion, it can easily be removed. A second guide wire is placed eccentrically into the condylar fragment to prevent rotation during reaming and insertion of the screw. After the two guide wires are placed, the skin is nicked

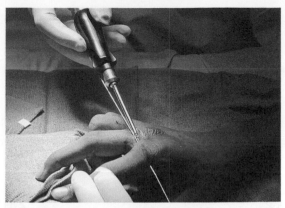

Fig. 4. The guide wire exits the opposite side of the digit so in case it breaks, it can be easily retrieved. The skin is nicked with the tip of an 11 blade, and the near cortex is hand reamed.

with the tip of an 11 blade over the central guide wire and blunt dissection with a hemostat is continued to the level of the bone surface.

In unicondylar fractures that involve soft metaphysial bone, only the near cortex needs to be reamed with the recently reduced self-drilling headless cannulated screws (**Fig. 4**). Typically, the screw length measures 8 to 10 mm. Under fluoroscopic control, the selected screw is placed dorsally outside the skin over the fracture site. The ideal length is selected and the screw is inserted over the guide wire so that it fits entirely inside the bone on the PA and lateral radiographs (**Figs. 5** and **6**).

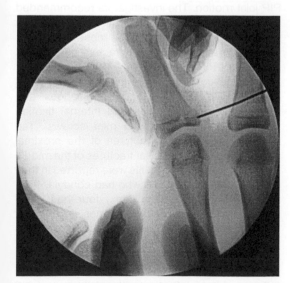

Fig. 3. A guide wire is inserted under fluoroscopy across the fracture site.

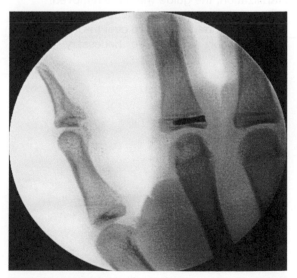

Fig. 5. Posteroanterior fluoroscopic view of a micro Acutrak II (Acumed, Hillsboro, Oregon) inserted over the guide wire anatomically reducing and stabilizing the fracture fragment.

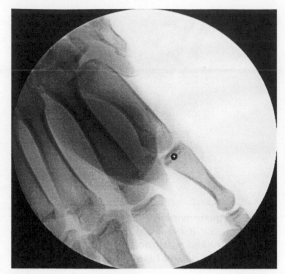

Fig. 6. Lateral radiograph of the headless cannulated screw in place securing the intraarticular fracture.

Occasionally, the condylar fragment extends proximally. In this instance, a second headless cannulated screw may be placed. The second mini screw is usually inserted on the opposite side from the first screw because of the obliquity of the fracture line. This placement allows the smaller diameter lead portion of the screw to cross the fracture site and engage the smaller remaining cortex of the condylar fragment decreasing the risk of fragmentation during insertion of the screw. The final mini screw position is fluoroscopically confirmed in the lateral and PA views. Following stabilization, the guide wires are removed.

The technique is percutaneous and only a small adhesive bandage is placed over the insertion site. No splint or sutures are necessary (**Fig. 7**).

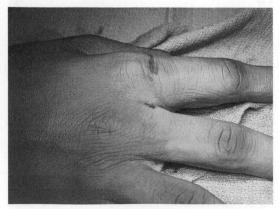

Fig. 7. The small incision needed to insert the screw. The skin is not closed with suture, and a band aid is placed over the small incision.

Immediate range-of-motion exercises are initiated, and strengthening exercises typically started 4 to 6 weeks following surgery. Athletes can return to competitive athletics within 1 week with the finger buddy-taped to the adjacent digit in a skilled player.

Intraarticular phalangeal base fractures may also be stabilized with one or more headless cannulated screws. Initial reduction is performed as previously described. The guide wire is inserted into the condylar fragment and advanced across the fracture to the opposite cortex of the phalanx parallel to the joint surface. A second derotation guide wire is placed eccentrically to prevent rotation of the condylar fragment as the headless cannulated screw is being inserted. A single mini screw provides sufficient stability for return to sports in most cases.

Weiss and Hastings reported on 38 consecutive distal unicondylar fractures of the proximal phalanx.[12] The average age of the patients was 24 years. There were 28 men. Fracture fixation included mini screws in 10 patients, mini screw and Kirschner wire in four patients, a single Kirschner wire fixation in 10 fractures, multiple Kirschner wires in 11 fractures, and loop wire fixation in one fracture. The fractures healed in all patients. The average proximal interphalangeal joint extension lag was 13 degrees (range 0–35 degrees) and PIP joint flexion averaged 85 degrees (range 60–115 degrees). They found that all four patients treated initially with single Kirschner wire fixation required a secondary procedure due to early fracture displacement. The group of patients whose condylar fracture was treated using two or more Kirschner wires ultimately had the best average PIP joint motion. The investigators recommended multiple Kirschner wire stabilization or mini screw fixation for those injuries as the most predictable method for achieving reliable fracture healing and recovery of PIP joint motion.

Ford and colleagues[15] reported a series of 36 patients with fractures of the phalanges and underwent open reduction and internal fixation with 1.5- and 2.0-mm AO mini screws. Ten patients had condylar fractures of the proximal phalanx and 4 had condylar fractures of the middle phalanx. No excellent results were reported in their series. Of the 10 patients who had condylar fractures of the proximal phalanx, four had good results and six had poor outcomes. In the four patients who had condylar fractures of the middle phalanx, two had good results and two had poor results. The investigators noted the tendency for the PIP joint to lose 20 to 30 degrees of extension following internal fixation with mini screws. PIP joint flexion was more reliably restored.

Geissler reported on 25 patients stabilized with percutaneous headless cannulated screw fixation for unicondylar fractures.[14] Eighteen patients had unicondylar fractures of the phalanx, three had intra-articular displaced fractures of the base of the phalanx, and four had intraarticular fractures along the base of the distal phalanx of the thumb. The fractures healed in all patients. There was no fracture displacement or malunion. No patients required screw removal. In the condylar phalangeal fractures, the average PIP joint loss of extension was 5 degrees (range 0–10 degrees) and the average PIP joint flexion was 85 degrees (range 80–95 degrees). In the four patients who had intra-articular fractures involving the base of the thumb, the average interphalangeal joint extension was 15 degrees (range 10–20 degrees), and the average flexion was 60 degrees (range 55–65 degrees). Geissler concluded that percutaneous fixation is less traumatic compared with open stabilization. Percutaneous cannulated mini screws retain the same advantage as percutaneous Kirschner wires and have the additional advantage of compressing the fracture site allowing more intensive and accelerated rehabilitation during the healing process. As the headless cannulated screw fits entirely within the bone, the implant is less likely to cause soft tissue irritation, does not migrate, and concern about pin track infection is eliminated compared with Kirschner wires.

PHALANGEAL SHAFT FRACTURES

Although percutaneous headless screw fixation is useful in unicondylar fractures and simple phalangeal shaft fractures, plate fixation may be required in athletes who have multiple fractures, comminution of the fracture site, and early return to athletic competition needs to be considered. In these instances, plate fixation is recommended. Plate fixation allows for immediate stability and active range of motion. Plate fixation also allows for immediate return to competition with protective bracing. Plates may be placed on the lateral or dorsal surface of the phalanx. It is the author's personal preference to place the plate on the lateral position of the phalanx. This placement potentially decreases adhesions from plate fixation secondary to the extensor digitorum communis tendon. The addition of the newer generation low-profile locking plates may further decrease the risk of tendon adhesions and promotes early range of motion.

The potential for high complication rates with plate fixation of the phalangeal shaft relates to the anatomy of the flexor and extensor tendons around the phalanges. In particular, the extensor mechanism covers the phalanges intimately and scarring of the extensor mechanism can occur not only from trauma in the fracture itself but also secondary to the approach required for plate fixation. Tendon gliding may be affected significantly in contrast to the metacarpals when there is more space available between the extensor tendons and the bone to accommodate plate stabilization.

However, this risk of scarring may be decreased in the collegiate athlete compared with the traditional patient. Under the close supervision of athletic trainers and physical therapy staff, the collegiate athlete may have access to physical therapy twice a day compared with the traditional patient who may receive therapy three times a week. This easy access to unlimited physical therapy allows the option of plate stabilization of phalangeal fractures with decreased risk of adhesions compared with traditional patients with limited access to physical therapy.

In the lateral approach, an incision is made in the mid axial line along the phalanx (**Figs. 8** and **9**). Blunt dissection is carried down to protect the cutaneous nerves, which are identified on the dorsal aspect of the wound. The volar aspect of the lateral band and the extensor digitorum communis tendon are retracted dorsally (**Fig. 10**). In fractures involving the base of the proximal phalanx, a portion of the lateral band may be excised. Depending on the fracture pattern, if one can choose either the radial or ulnar side of

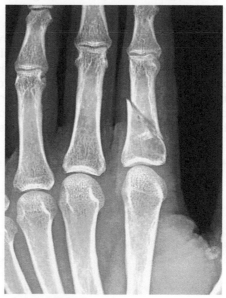

Fig. 8. Posteroanterior radiograph of a displaced phalangeal fracture of the proximal phalanx to the index finger in a collegiate starting defensive back.

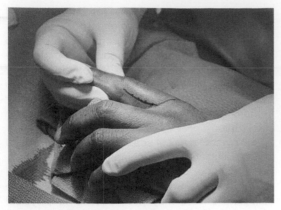

Fig. 9. A lateral approach to the index finger is made. Preferably, the incision is made on the ulnar side of the digit so as not to affect the lumbrical intrinsic insertion to the lateral band.

the digit, the ulnar side should be selected for the approach so as not to affect the lumbrical insertion onto the lateral band. The lateral band and extensor digitorum communis tendon are elevated and retracted dorsally exposing the fracture site (**Fig. 11**). A low-profile locking plate is placed on the side of the phalanx and locking and nonlocking screws are placed. Initially, nonlocking screws are placed to reduce the plate to the bone so there is no gap. Nonlocking lag screws are placed across the fracture site through the plate (**Fig. 12**). Locking screws are placed after the fracture is reduced and the plate is firmly against the bone surface (**Fig. 13**). The wound is closed in layers.

Long oblique fractures (fracture length is twice or greater than the diameter of the bone) may also be treated occasionally with headless mini screw fixation when immediate return to competition is not an issue. Manipulative reduction similar to the technique for condylar fractures is performed. Pointed reduction forceps provide provisional stabilization after the fracture is anatomically reduced under fluoroscopic control on the PA and lateral views. Guide wires are

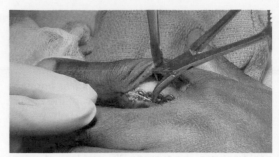

Fig. 11. A Medartis (Basel, Switzerland) 2.0 locking plate is placed on the ulnar side of the proximal phalanx.

placed across the fracture fragment exiting the skin on the opposite side of the digit. Fracture reduction and position of the guide wires is confirmed fluoroscopically. In this instance, the cortical bone is quite rigid compared with the softer metaphyseal bone. Because of this, the near and far cortex are reamed. This procedure significantly decreases the risk of the opposite cortex being blown out by insertion of the headless cannulated screw. Following reaming of the cortical bone, the headless cannulated screws are inserted so that the widest parts of the screws are positioned opposite each other to allow maximum bone purchase. Frequently, the screws are placed in opposite directions. Percutaneous stabilization decreases the risk of adhesions and promotes an improved range of motion.

Dabezies and Schutte reported good results in 22 patients who underwent plate fixation of proximal phalangeal fractures.[15] In their study, the patients had an average total active motion of 243 degrees maintaining an average total active motion of 247 degrees. Stiffness of the metacarpal

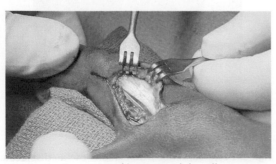

Fig. 10. The lateral band is retracted dorsally to expose the fracture site.

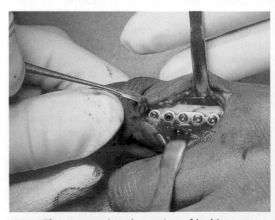

Fig. 12. The surgeon has the option of locking or nonlocking screws to stabilize the fracture. Nonlocking screws are potentially used to lag across the fracture site through the plate.

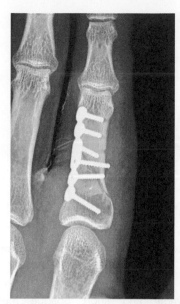

Fig. 13. Posteroanterior radiograph showing anatomic restoration and stability to the fracture site. With plate fixation, the athlete is allowed to return to competition within a few weeks.

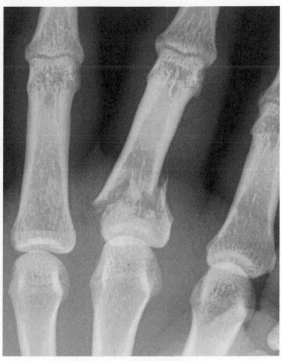

Fig. 15. Posteroanterior radiograph showing a displaced fracture to the base of the proximal phalanx on the long finger.

phalangeal joint or proximal phalangeal joint was noted in only two cases. Bosscha and Snellen reported that 6 of 7 phalangeal fractures regained total active motion greater than 220 degrees, stabilized by plate fixation.[16] Berman and colleagues noted that good and excellent results were achieved in 94% of 16 patients who underwent plate stabilization of the phalangeal fracture.

However, Page and Stern showed that only 11% of 37 phalangeal fractures treated with plate stabilization regained total active motion greater than 220 degrees, and 92% of these fractures had

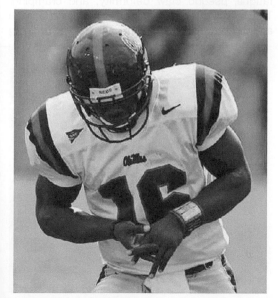

Fig. 14. Starting Ole Miss quarterback with an obvious deformity to the proximal phalanx of his long finger on his throwing hand.

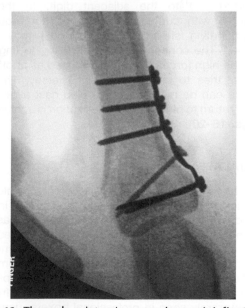

Fig. 16. Through a lateral approach, a mini fixation plate is placed along the lateral border of the digit anatomically reducing and stabilizing the fracture.

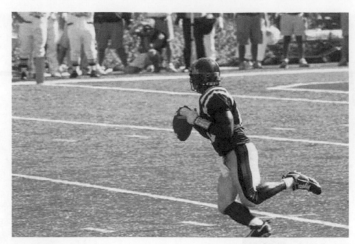

Fig. 17. The Ole Miss quarterback released to return to play within 2 weeks, preparing to throw a touchdown pass with a specialized playing splint.

one or more complications including extensor lag (59.5%), contracture (37.8%), delayed union (2.7%), and plate prominence (2.7%).[17]

However, these complications can be minimized by low-profile locking plates placed on the radial or ulnar side of the phalanx and not directly underneath the extensor tendon on the dorsal surface. In addition, the high performance collegiate athlete has the advantage of exposure to physical therapy once or twice a day, which can minimize the complications of stiffness.

Depending on the athlete's position, the patient is returned to athletics (**Figs. 14–17**). In patients who have a skilled position, the athlete's finger is buddy-taped to the adjacent digit. In those athletes with contact and who do not require ball-handling skills, a club-type cast may be placed. The concern is not a blow to the finger, but the high forces that are introduced as another player tries to grab the patient's jersey. These forces can be minimized by a club cast allowing early return to play when stable fixation is achieved (**Figs. 18–20**).

METACARPAL FRACTURES

Fractures of the metacarpal are common athletic injuries, particularly in contact sports. The incidence of metacarpal fractures generally increases toward the ulnar side of the hand with fractures of the fifth metacarpal being the most common. Metacarpal neck fractures are the most common and usually involve the ring and small metacarpals. However, metacarpal neck fractures (boxer's fractures), rarely seen in professional boxers, usually occur in amateur boxers who hit solid objects and in street brawlers.

Transverse and short oblique metacarpal fractures tend to angle dorsally because of the deforming forces of the intrinsic flexors and intrinsic musculature on the distal fragment. Most metacarpal shaft and subcapital fractures present with a dorsal angulation deformity. As much as 7 degrees of extensor lag and 8% loss of grip strength have been shown to occur for each 2 mm of metacarpal shortening.[18–20] Intrinsic muscle shortening and altered muscle tension may lead to progressive measurable grip strength weakness after approximately 30 degrees of dorsal metacarpal angulation.[18] Athletes may complain of loss of knuckle contour, muscle fatigue, pseudo claw deformity, and cramping. The border metacarpals (index and small) have an inherent tendency for greater shortening

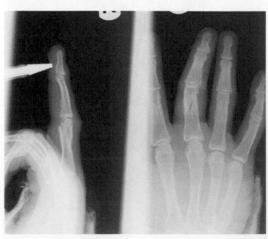

Fig. 18. Posteroanterior and lateral radiographs of a displaced unstable fracture to the proximal phalanx in the starting Ole Miss linebacker.

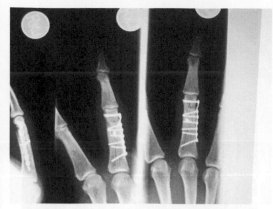

Fig. 19. The fracture was stabilized with a mini fixation plate situated on the lateral border of the proximal phalanx to the long finger.

compared with the long and ring metacarpals due to lack of support of the deep intermetacarpal ligaments. Border metacarpals have a greater tolerance for lateral angulation compared with the long and ring metacarpals because of the greater divergence as they have only one adjacent finger. Rotation of the metacarpals is poorly tolerated. Each degree of metacarpal fracture rotation may produce as much as 5 degrees of rotation at the fingertips.[21] It has been shown that approximately 10 degrees of metacarpal rotation will result in 2 cm of fingertip overlap.[21] Clinical deformity from lateral metacarpal angulation is best observed with the finger straight, whereas a rotational deformity is best observed with the fingers in flexion.

METACARPAL HEAD FRACTURES

It is controversial how much angulation to accept in metacarpal neck fractures involving the ring

and small metacarpals. Ford and colleagues reviewed 62 fractures of the small metacarpal neck and concluded that a palm angulation of 70 degrees resulted in good outcomes.[22] In their study, the fracture was not reduced and the hand was immobilized. Eichenholtz and colleagues[23] considered that palmar angulation more than 40 degrees required correction. Other investigators have recommended operative intervention if there is angulation greater than 30 degrees.[24] If a rotation or clawing deformity is noted to the small or ring metacarpal, then reduction and stabilization should be considered. Due to the more rigid index and long carpal metacarpal joints, angulation of up to only 10 degrees may be acceptable for fractures involving the index and long metacarpals.

Several methods of fixation have been recommended for metacarpal neck fractures. These include transverse pinning of the metacarpal head into the adjacent metacarpal and intramedullary pinning. These techniques are particularly more cosmetic in the female patient who is concerned about a scar. For fractures that involve comminution, plate fixation with a mini condylar plate or T plate may be an option. The advantage of plate fixation allows early return to competition and rehabilitation compared with protruding Kirschner wire stabilization. As described earlier, the metacarpals are not as closely surrounded by the extensor tendons, which allows more forgiveness for a metal implant, particularly with the newer generation of low-profile locking plates.

METACARPAL SHAFT FRACTURES

Most isolated metacarpal shaft fractures are stable. Border metacarpal fractures are less stable due to the lack of adjacent soft tissue support.

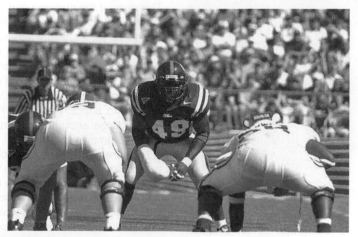

Fig. 20. The starting Ole Miss linebacker clear to return to play within a week in a club cast, preparing to make a tackle on an opposing player.

Transverse fractures have a tendency to angulate and apex dorsally due to the pull of the intrinsic musculature and the extrinsic flexor tendons. Due to the mobility of the hamate saddle joint, up to 20 degrees of angulation is acceptable for transverse shaft fractures of the small and ring metacarpals. Due to the lack of mobility of the index and long metacarpals at the carpal metacarpal joint, only 5 to 10 degrees of angulation may be accepted in the index and long metacarpals.

Plate fixation should be considered in contact athletes when return to competition as soon as possible is desired. For the metacarpals, 2-mm plates are recommended with four cortices proximal and distal to the fracture site for adequate fracture stability. Newer generation locking cage plates are strong and provide multiple screw fixation in a short distance and are useful particularly when metacarpal comminution is present (**Figs. 21** and **22**). In the contact sport athlete, the patient will be cleared to return to play within the first few weeks wearing a fracture brace when it is felt that adequate fracture stability has been achieved with plate fixation.

Oblique metacarpal fractures have a tendency to shorten along the oblique slope of the fracture line, particularly in the index and small metacarpals due to the lack of support of the deep transverse metacarpal ligament. Frequently, in an oblique fracture pattern, the fracture line is too short for lag screw fixation alone and a single lag screw needs to be neutralized by a plate. It is recommended that 2.0- or 1.5-mm screws and a plate are used. The fracture is compressed by the lag screw and once fracture stability is achieved,

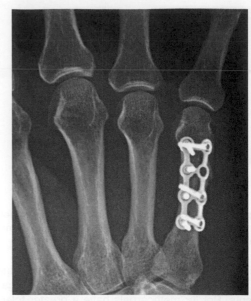

Fig. 22. The fracture was stabilized with a Medartis (Basel, Switzerland) cage plate. The cage plate provides sufficient stability to allow the player to return early to competition.

a T plate or L plate is then placed on the dorsum of the metacarpal.

When considering the use of lag screw fixation to stabilize a bone fragment, the fracture fragment should be at least three times the diameter of the screw. During open reduction, stabilization with a screw is preferable to a Kirschner wire. The advantage of a screw over a wire is that it can compress the fracture to provide additional stability. If the fragment is large enough to place a Kirschner wire, it is usually large enough to accept a screw for compression. A 0.45 Kirschner wire is equal to the diameter of a 1.1-mm drill bit. Therefore, if the surgeon can get a 0.45 Kirschner into a small bone fragment, this is the same size as the drill bit for a 1.5-mm screw. The Kirschner wire can be removed and fixation would be improved by addition of a 1.5-mm compression screw. Similarly, a 0.065 Kirschner wire is equal in diameter to a 1.5-mm drill bit. If the fracture fragment is large enough to support a 0.065 Kirschner wire, it is usually large enough for fixation with a 2.0-mm screw for improved stability.

Lag screws are the implant choice for spiral fractures of the metacarpals when the fracture line is at least twice the diameter of the bone. A minimum of two screws is required. One screw may be placed perpendicular to the shaft, which helps with translation of the fracture, and a second screw is placed perpendicular to the fracture line to compress the fracture. Alternatively, two screws may be placed

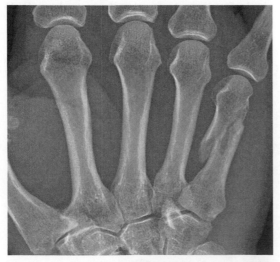

Fig. 21. Posteroanterior radiograph of an unstable fifth metacarpal fracture in a collegiate basketball player.

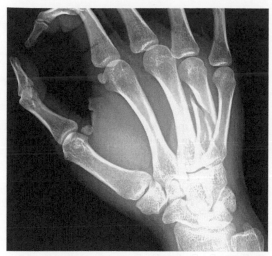

Fig. 23. Oblique radiograph showing an unstable fracture in a collegiate football player.

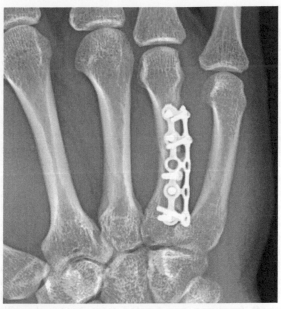

Fig. 25. Posteroanterior radiograph showing stabilization of the ring metacarpal fracture with a cage plate and lag screw fixation. The athlete was returned to play within a week following stabilization.

bisecting the angle of the fracture and the shaft. It is recommended that a 2.0- or 1.5-mm screw is used if lag screw fixation is used for a spiral metacarpal fracture.

Lag screw fixation offers the advantage of potentially less surgical dissection compared with application of a plate, which would result in less tendon adhesion and scarring. However, due to the increased distance of the extensor tendons from the metacarpal, plate fixation of

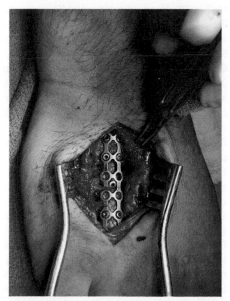

Fig. 24. The index metacarpal fracture is stabilized with a Medartis (Basel, Switzerland) cage plate. The cage plate allows for lag screw fixation between the screw holes to further stabilize the fracture.

metacarpals is well tolerated, and results in minimal scarring and decreased range of motion. Dabezies and Schutte reported their results for plating of 27 unstable metacarpal fractures (average total active motion of 252 degrees); they had 1 complication of metacarpophalangeal joint stiffness.[15] Bosscha and Snellen reported that 29 of 31 metacarpal fractures regained total active motion greater than 220 degrees.[16]

Geissler reviewed his results on open reduction and internal fixation of metacarpal phalangeal fractures in athletes.[25] Open reduction and internal fixation with a 2.0 locking cage plate was performed in 8 of 10 patients with fractures of the metacarpal (**Figs. 23–25**). Two patients underwent lag screw fixation for a spiral fracture of the metacarpal. Patients were allowed to return to competition between 1 and 2 weeks following fixation. The fractures healed in all patients in an acute postoperative period. One patient who had lag screw fixation of a spiral fracture to the index metacarpal sustained a refracture to the index metacarpal approximately 1 year following stabilization after sliding into a base during a baseball game. The report on his injury concluded that although lag screws are certainly the implant of choice in long, spiral metacarpal fractures, plate fixation needs to be considered, particularly in the border digits of metacarpal fractures in contact athletes.

SUMMARY

Metacarpal and phalangeal fractures are common athletic injuries. These injuries can significantly affect the athlete's career particularly when they occur during the athlete's playing season. It also can significantly affect the athlete's training when these injuries occur in the off season. For this reason, stable fixation is recommended in those patients with displaced and unstable fracture patterns. Unicondylar phalangeal fractures are inherently unstable, and operative fixation is recommended. Percutaneous insertion of headless cannulated screws offers several advantages compared with traditional mini screw fixation and Kirschner wires. Headless cannulated mini screws do not protrude from the bone and are less likely to impale or impinge on the collateral ligaments. Percutaneous insertion causes minimal scarring and potentially improves the range of motion in this complicated injury. Most unstable phalangeal shaft fractures are treated percutaneously with Kirschner wire fixation to minimize scarring. However, in the contact athlete who desires early return to competition, or in comminuted fracture patterns, plate fixation is an option. In this instance, it is recommended that the plate be placed on the radial or ulnar border of the phalanx to avoid scarring from the closely adhered extensor tendon on the dorsal aspect of the phalanx. Particularly in collegiate athletes who have the advantage of aggressive daily physical therapy, stiffness secondary to scarring can be minimized.

Plate fixation of unstable metacarpal fractures is better tolerated with a decreased risk of stiffness compared with the phalanges due to the increased distance of the extensor tendon mechanism from the bone. Kirschner wire fixation or intramedullary fixation is an option particularly in patients for whom cosmesis is important. However, for the athletes who desire early return to competition or training, plate fixation is recommended. Plate fixation is also suggested for contact athletes who have a long spiral fracture, particularly in the border digits, rather than lag screw fixation, to decrease the potential complication of refracture on a lag screw.

REFERENCES

1. Green DP, Rowland SA. Fractures and dislocations in the hand. In: Rockwood CA Jr, Green DP, Bucholz RW, editors. Fractures in adults, vol. 1, 3rd edition. Philadelphia: Lippincott; 1991. p. 441.
2. Kelsey JL, Pastides H, Kreiger N, et al. Upper extremity disorders: a survey of their frequency, impact, and cost in the United States. St. Louis (MO): Mosby; 1997. p. 9–71.
3. Hove LM. Fractures of the hand. Distribution and relative incidence. Scand J Plast Reconstr Surg 1993;27(4):317–9.
4. Emmett JE, Breck LW. A review and analysis of 11,000 fractures seen in a private practice of orthopaedic surgery, 1937–1956. J Bone Joint Surg Am 1958;40(5):1169–75.
5. de Jonge JJ, Kingma J, van der Lei B, et al. Fractures of the metacarpals: a retrospective analysis of incidence and etiology and a review of the English language literature. Injury 1994;25(6):365–9.
6. Chung KC, Spilson SV. The frequency and epidemiology of hand and forearm fractures in the United States. J Hand Surg Am 2001;26(5):908–15.
7. Belsky MR, Eaton RG, Lane LB. Closed reduction and internal fixation of proximal phalangeal fractures. J Hand Surg Am 1984;9(5):725–9.
8. Eaton R, Burton R. Fractures of the hand. In: Kilgore ES Jr, Graham WP, editors. The hand: surgical and non-surgical management. Philadelphia: Lea & Febiger; 1977. p. 121–42.
9. Stern PJ. Management of fractures of the hand over the last 25 years. J Hand Surg Am 2000;25(5): 817–23.
10. London PS. Sprains and fractures involving the interphalangeal joints. Hand 1971;3(2):155–8.
11. Stark HH. Troublesome fractures and dislocations of the hand. In: Lovell WW, MacAusland WR, Stamp WG, editors. AAOS instructional course lectures. St. Louis (MO): Mosby; 1970. p. 130–49.
12. Weiss AP, Hastings H 2nd. Distal unicondylar fractures of the proximal phalanx. J Hand Surg Am 1993;18(4):594–9.
13. McCue FC, Honner R, Johnson MC, et al. Athletic injuries of the proximal interphalangeal joint requiring surgical treatment. J Bone Joint Surg Am 1970;52(5): 937–56.
14. Geissler WB. Cannulated percutaneous fixation of intra-articular hand fractures. In: Freeland AE, Lindley SG, editors. Hand clinics. Hand fractures and dislocations, WB Saunders Company, Philadelphia, vol. 22(3) 2006:297–305.
15. Dabezies EJ, Schutte JP. Fixation of metacarpal and phalangeal fractures with miniature plate and screws. J Hand Surg Am 1986;11(2):283–8.
16. Bosscha K, Snellen JP. Internal fixation of metacarpal and phalangeal fractures with AO minifragment screws and plates: a prospective study. Injury 1993;24(3):166–8.
17. Berman KS, Rothkopf DM, Shufflebarger JV, et al. Internal fixation of phalangeal fractures using titanium miniplates. Ann Plast Surg 1999;42(4):408–10.
18. Low CK, Wong HC, Low YP, et al. A cadaver study of the effects of dorsal angulation and shortening of the metacarpal shaft on the extension and flexion force ratios of the index and little fingers. J Hand Surg Br 1995;20(5):609–13.

19. Meunier MJ, Hentzen E, Ryan M, et al. Predicted effects of metacarpal shortening on interosseous muscle function. J Hand Surg Am 2004;29(4):689–93.

20. Strauch RJ, Rosenwasser MP, Lunt JG. Metacarpal shaft fractures: the effect of shortening on the extensor tendon mechanism. J Hand Surg [Am] 1998;23(3):519–23.

21. Royle SG. Rotational deformity following metacarpal fracture. J Hand Surg Br 1990;15(1):124–5.

22. Ford D, Ali M, Steel WM. Fractures of the fifth metacarpal neck: is reduction or immobilization necessary? J Hand Surg Br 1989;14:165–7.

23. Eichenholz S, Yonkers N, Rizzo P. Fracture of the neck of the fifth metacarpal bone: is overtreatment justified? JAMA 1961;178:425–6.

24. Stern PJ. Fractures of the metacarpals and phalanges. In: Green DP, Hotchkiss RN, Pederson WC, editors. Green's operative hand surgery. 4th edition. New York: Churchill Livingstone; 1999. p. 711–71.

25. Geissler WB, McCraney WO. Operative management of metacarpal fractures. In: Ring DC, Cohen MS, editors. Fractures of the hand and wrist. New York: Informa Healthcare USA, Inc.; 2007. p. 75–89.

Management of Proximal Interphalangeal Joint Dislocations in Athletes

Randy R. Bindra, MD, FRCS*, Brian J. Foster, MD

KEYWORDS

- Proximal interphalangeal joint
- Dislocation • Fracture • Pilon • Volar plate

Proximal interphalangeal joint dislocations are common injuries in athletes. These injuries may be associated with fractures of the base of the middle phalanx. Principles of management include achieving and maintaining a congruent joint, early mobilization to prevent stiffness, and restoration of the joint articular surface, which is the least important issue. An athlete or coach may minimize injury to the proximal interphalangeal joint, especially dislocations that are reduced on the field; therefore, it is the responsibility of the treating orthopedic surgeon to fully and carefully evaluate and treat these injuries. In the following sections, basic anatomy, injury pathology and characteristics, clinical assessment, radiological findings, and treatment principles are reviewed.

ANATOMY

The proximal interphalangeal (PIP) joint is a hinge joint that accounts for 85% of the motion required to grasp an object.[1] The PIP joint is formed by proximal and middle phalanges and derives its stability from its bony architecture and soft tissue restraints. The majority of joint motion is in flexion-extension, with a normal range of motion between 100° and 120°. The proximal phalanx head has two concentric condyles that are separated by an intercondylar concavity or notch. The condyles articulate with corresponding concavities on the broad base of the middle phalanx.

These concavities are separated by a saddle-shaped median ridge; the ridge fits into the corresponding intercondylar notch of the proximal phalanx for bony stability. This congruence offers stability in flexion-extension while limiting lateral and rotational movements.[2]

A collateral ligament on each lateral aspect of the PIP joint limits radial and ulnar deviation and offers side-to-side stability (**Fig. 1**). The ligaments arise from a notch distal to the epicondyle of the proximal phalanx and run in an oblique and volar direction to insert onto the middle phalanx in its volar lateral aspect. Each collateral ligament has two parts: a dorsal component that tightens during flexion and a volar component that tightens in extension.[3] A separate accessory collateral ligament runs with each proper collateral ligament; however, this accessory collateral ligament runs in a more volar direction to insert on the lateral edge of the volar plate and flexor tendon sheath. The primary function of the accessory ligament is to tension the volar plate and pull it proximally to provide clearance during finger flexion.[4]

Spanning the volar aspect of the joint is the volar plate, which primarily prevents hyperextension of the joint.[4] The volar plate is secured proximally to the proximal phalanx through thick lateral extensions (checkrein ligaments) that attach to the bone within the distal aspect of the second annular pulley. The proximal edge of the plate remains free so that it can move proximally during digital flexion. Its proximal origins are also confluent

Department of Orthopaedic Surgery, Loyola University Medical Center, Maguire Center Suite 1700, 2160 South 1st Avenue, Maywood, IL 60153, USA

* Corresponding author.

E-mail address: rbindra@lumc.edu (R.R. Bindra).

Hand Clin 25 (2009) 423–435
doi:10.1016/j.hcl.2009.05.008
0749-0712/09/$ – see front matter © 2009 Elsevier Inc. All rights reserved.

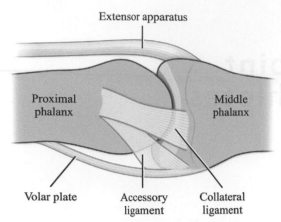

Extensor apparatus

Proximal phalanx

Middle phalanx

Volar plate

Accessory ligament

Collateral ligament

Fig. 1. Key anatomic structures surrounding the PIP joint.

with the proximal origins of the first cruciate pulley. The volar plate's central distal attachment is to the base of the middle phalanx where it blends with the periosteum just volar to the articular surface; its lateral distal attachment is thicker and blends with the insertion of the collateral ligaments. The volar plate and collateral ligaments form a strong boxlike design that stabilizes the PIP joint and resists joint displacement. PIP joint displacement occurs when the ligament-box complex is disrupted in at least two planes.[3,5] The volar plate and accessory collateral ligaments maintain joint stability in the extended PIP joint whereas the proper collateral ligaments maintain stability in flexion.[3]

The flexor and extensor tendons provide additional stability. The central slip of the extensor mechanism crosses over the PIP joint before it attaches to the dorsum of the middle phalanx. The lateral bands of the extensor mechanism (composed of the lumbrial and dorsal interossei tendons) travel on both sides of the PIP joint; they are held in place over the PIP joint by the transverse retinacular ligament. The flexor tendons are held close to the volar aspect of the joint by the third annular pulley, which attaches to the volar plate. In addition, the flexor digitorum superficialis tendon directly inserts on either side of the volar lateral edge of the middle phalanx through two lateral slips.

The PIP joint dorsal capsule has a small synovial lining and is separate from the overlying extensor mechanism.[6] The volar capsule consists of the volar plate, the proximal extension of which is continuous with a band of connective tissue that extends to the proximal phalanx neck.[2] The radial and ulnar aspects of the joint capsule can each be divided into three components: the collateral ligament and the two fan-shaped areas dorsal and

volar to it. The fibers of the dorsal fan-shaped area blend distally with the extensor expansion; the fibers of the volar fan-shaped area blend distally with the collateral ligament, volar plate, and flexor sheath.[2]

INJURY CHARACTERISTICS

Due to its unprotected location, long lever arm, and low lateral and rotational mobility, the PIP joint is susceptible to injury in athletes.[7] Athletes who participate in sports involving catching or hitting a ball are especially susceptible to PIP injuries. Many of these injuries occur from the athlete "jamming" or "catching" their finger while catching a ball or falling, resulting in hyperextension or angular deformity to the PIP joint. Compounding the actual injury, the PIP joint has a propensity for stiffness after trauma or immobilization, especially immobilization of longer than 3 weeks.[8] This stiffness is likely due to pain, swelling, and fibrosis/scar tissue formation.

PIP injuries include sprains, dislocations, and fracture-dislocations. PIP dislocations are identified by the direction of the middle phalanx in relation to the proximal phalanx. If associated with fractures of the base of the middle phalanx, they are classified as fracture-dislocations. Increasing instability is associated with increased size of fracture fragments. The three types of PIP dislocations are dorsal (most common), volar, and lateral. The volar plate and at least one collateral ligament must be injured for PIP dislocation to occur.

PROXIMAL INTERPHALANGEAL JOINT DORSAL DISLOCATIONS

By far the most common type of PIP dislocation, dorsal dislocations, occur secondary to hyperextension of the PIP joint; there is usually also an axial load component to the deforming force. In these injuries, the volar plate is avulsed from the middle phalanx base and the middle phalanx rests on the dorsum of the proximal phalanx. The middle phalanx is dislocated dorsally and the volar plate is avulsed from its distal insertion, thus helping to prevent the plate from incarcerating within the joint. The volar plate usually retains its proximal and lateral attachments to the proximal phalanx and accessory collateral ligament, respectively.[4]

Dorsal PIP dislocations occur along a spectrum of injuries to the PIP joint. As a result of hyperextension injury, most injuries result in avulsion of the volar plate at its distal attachment with or without a small bony fragment. The collateral ligaments remain intact and joint congruity is maintained; clinically this presents as a "sprained" joint. With more severe applied force, in addition to volar plate avulsion, the collateral ligaments split longitudinally allowing dorsal dislocation of the middle phalanx (**Fig. 2**). The most severe form of injury is one resulting from hyperextension and axial loading, resulting in dorsal PIP dislocation with a shear fracture of the volar lip of the middle phalanx as it makes contact with the head of the proximal phalanx. With larger fracture fragments involving more than 40% of the articular surface of the middle phalanx, the dorsal fragment is bereft of any stabilizing soft tissue attachment as the volar plate and collateral ligaments remain with the volar fracture fragment (**Fig. 3**).[5,9] The additional loss of bony congruity creates an extremely unstable situation whereby it is difficult to maintain joint reduction.

PROXIMAL INTERPHALANGEAL JOINT LATERAL DISLOCATIONS

A laterally directed force to the PIP joint results in avulsion of the collateral ligament from its proximal attachment on the side of the applied force (**Fig. 4**).[7,10] With continued force the volar plate eventually tears on the side of injury, resulting in lateral dislocation.

PROXIMAL INTERPHALANGEAL JOINT VOLAR DISLOCATIONS

Volar PIP dislocations are rare and unlike the more common dorsal or lateral dislocations, are

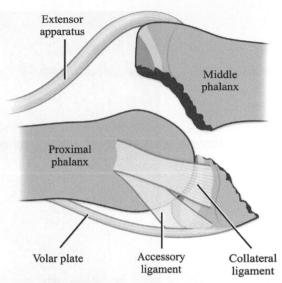

Fig. 3. Anatomic features of a dorsal PIP fracture-dislocation with a fracture fragment consisting of more than 40% of the middle phalanx base. The loss of bony congruity along with disruption of all ligamentous stabilizers creates an extremely unstable configuration.

sometimes irreducible due to soft tissue interposition.[11] In uncomplicated cases the central slip of the extensor mechanism ruptures or avulses from the dorsal lip of the middle phalanx (**Fig. 5**).[10] The intact lateral bands initially can perform joint extension even though the central slip is ruptured. Failure to immobilize the joint in extension to allow central slip healing can eventually lead to stretching of the triangular ligament holding the lateral bands, resulting in their volar subluxation. The subluxated lateral bands can no longer extend the PIP joint and the tightening of the terminal extensor slip leads to hyperextension of the distal interphalangeal (DIP) joint: the classic boutonniere deformity.

Complex volar dislocations involve rotary displacement with a collateral ligament tear secondary to lateral stress combined with an anteriorly directed force. In complicated cases the central slip, lateral band, or torn collateral ligament may be interposed within the joint, thereby necessitating open reduction.[12]

PROXIMAL INTERPHALANGEAL JOINT FRACTURE-DISLOCATIONS

These injuries result in PIP dislocation with a fracture of the proximal base of the middle phalanx. Hyperextension or hyperflexion loads result in avulsion fractures, whereas axial loading in varying positions of PIP flexion/extension leads to

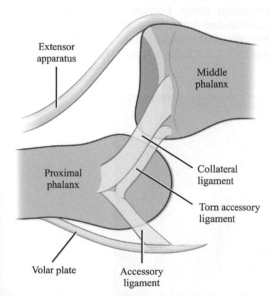

Fig. 2. Ligamentous injuries associated with a simple dorsal PIP dislocation. Apart from the volar plate and part of the accessory collateral ligament, other important structures and hence joint stability is preserved.

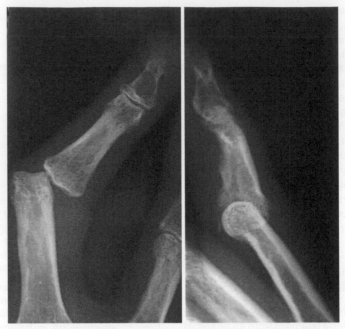

Fig. 4. Anteroposterior and lateral radiographs of a lateral dislocation of the PIP joint.

impaction shear fractures.[9,13] The fractures are located at one of three locations on the middle phalanx: volar lip, dorsal lip, or central (pilon fracture).

Avulsion fractures are either volar or dorsal and can involve varying amounts of the middle phalanx articular surface, although they generally involve less than a third of the articular surface. Tiny volar avulsion "chip" fractures are more common, represent an avulsion of the volar plate, and are secondary to a hyperextension injury. Dorsal avulsion fractures are less common and are secondary

to an axial force flexing an extended digit, thereby avulsing the central slip of the extensor mechanism. Impaction shear fractures have more comminution than avulsion fractures and occur when an axial stress is applied to the PIP joint in varying angles of flexion or extension. Axial stress in flexion produces a volar impaction shear fracture and stress in extension results in a dorsal impaction shear fracture.[13] Pilon fractures are comminuted fractures that result in fractures of the volar and dorsal cortices with compression of the central articular surface. These are secondary

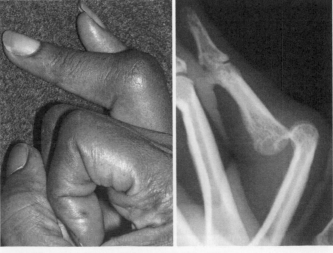

Fig. 5. Clinical and radiographic appearance of a volar PIP dislocation.

to axial load in neutral or hyperextension. The multiple small fracture fragments are often too small for fixation of all the fragments.

Because there is a correlation between the amount of articular surface that is fractured and PIP joint stability, PIP fracture-dislocations are generally classified based on the amount of articular surface involvement (ie, Grade I = 0%, Grade II = 0%–20%, and so forth).[5,9,14] However, their prognosis and treatment are best evaluated by simply labeling them as "stable" or "unstable" based on clinical and radiographic assessment. "Stable" volar lip fractures generally involve less than 30% of the articular surface and maintain joint reduction through a full arc of motion. "Unstable" volar lip fractures usually involve 40% to 50% of the articular surface and redislocate as the digit is moved into extension. More severe injuries generally are only stable in extreme degrees of flexion.

CLINICAL FEATURES

As with any sports injury, a thorough physical examination is important in a patient with a PIP joint injury. In addition to the physical examination, a detailed history including handedness, specific position or activity in sport, level of competition, status of the current sport season, and patient expectations and goals are important considerations. It is generally advisable to examine the unaffected digits, hand, and wrist before examining the PIP joint in question. Swelling, skin integrity, areas of tenderness, active and passive range of motion (ROM), and scissoring when the patient makes a fist should be noted. A dislocation can easily be determined clinically, but a minor subluxation may be more subtle and is suggested with severe restriction of PIP joint motion or scissoring. Although neurovascular injuries are uncommon in PIP injuries, capillary refill and two-point discrimination should be examined in the affected digits. Integrity of the central slip, flexor superficialis, and flexor profundus must be examined individually. Finally, ROM and stability of the adjacent joints in the same digit must be tested so that additional injuries in the same digit are not missed.

Further examination of joint stability is performed after closed reduction under local anesthetic is achieved. Stability testing should include taking the PIP joint through a full ROM of flexion-extension and side-side stressing. Radiographs should be obtained before any reduction, manipulation, or stability testing. Testing side-side joint stability with the joint fully extended and in 30° of flexion assesses collateral integrity. A laxity of 10° in extension and 20° in flexion indicates proper collateral ligament rupture; 15° laxity in extension and 30° in flexion indicate additional accessory collateral ligament rupture.[3] The joint is then moved through flexion-extension and the position of any recurrent subluxation or dislocation is recorded.

Some PIP joint dislocations may have been already been treated on the field and present after closed reduction. It is important to determine the direction of the previous deformity and perform a thorough physical examination, specifically assessing joint stability. Stability should be assessed after radiographs, as nondisplaced fracture fragments may move when manipulated under anesthesia. It is not uncommon to have associated injuries to the distal interphalangeal joint, especially mallet injuries as they have a common mechanism of injury. Clinical and radiographic evaluation must exclude associated injury to the DIP joint (**Fig. 6**).

IMAGING

Evaluation of PIP joint injuries demands thorough examination of accurate posteroanterior (PA), lateral, and oblique radiographs centered on the injured digit. It is important to obtain radiographs before reductions or stability testing. Postreduction radiographs should be carefully reviewed to ensure concentric joint reduction and look for any displaced or interposed fracture fragments. A true lateral view should reveal a congruent joint space with two parallel surfaces. PIP joint subluxation may be difficult to appreciate but can be represented on the lateral view by a "V" sign, which is divergence of the posterior articular surfaces from the central aspect of the joint (**Fig. 7**).[15] It is essential to confirm joint congruency on posteroanterior and lateral views immediately after reduction and serially during treatment.

MANAGEMENT OF PROXIMAL INTERPHALANGEAL JOINT DISLOCATIONS AND FRACTURE-DISLOCATIONS

The primary goal for treatment of PIP dislocations and fracture-dislocations is to restore joint alignment and maintain joint stability so that the patient can perform early ROM exercises. Early ROM has a positive effect on cartilage and soft tissue healing, and decreases adhesions. The middle phalanx must glide around the head of the proximal phalanx during flexion instead of hinging at the fracture margin; joint subluxation prevents gliding.[9] The secondary goal of treatment is to maintain articular congruity, although this can be sacrificed to achieve joint stability and early ROM.

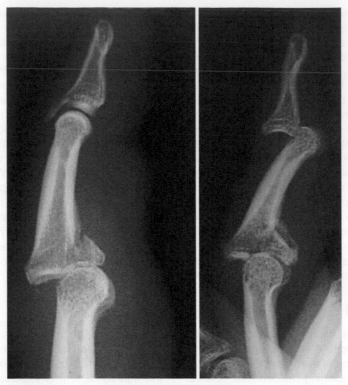

Fig. 6. Radiographs demonstrating concurrent PIP and DIP joint injuries. The radiograph on the left shows a dorsal PIP fracture-dislocation with bony mallet finger. On the right the finger shows a PIP pilon fracture associated with a DIP dislocation.

Most dislocations and stable fractures can be treated conservatively with closed reduction and early ROM. Anatomic studies have shown that on reduction of dorsolateral PIP dislocations, the injured volar plate and collateral ligaments return to their anatomic positions.[16] Injuries that fail conservative treatment or are unstable require more aggressive management, such as percutaneous fixation or traction. Open reduction internal fixation (ORIF) is not frequently required and is usually used in the treatment of injuries that present late. Athletes must be treated in the context of their sport. It is vital to take into account the athlete's specific sport, level of competition, position/role, future requirements, and goals/expectations.

CONSERVATIVE MANAGEMENT
Dorsal Proximal Interphalangeal Dislocations

If seen within a few days of injury, most dorsal PIP dislocations can be treated with closed reduction. Closed reduction of dorsal PIP dislocations is performed after digital block is administered. Gentle longitudinal traction is applied followed by flexion at the PIP joint. Joint stability is tested after reduction and while the digital block is still in effect. As long as the PIP joint is stable, small volar lip

avulsion fractures do not require specific management and the digit is mobilized with buddy taping to an adjacent digit to prevent hyperextension for 3 weeks. There is no need to splint in flexion, as this can lead to flexion contractures. Athletes may return to their sport with buddy tapping as symptoms allow. Active and passive ROM should be started as soon as possible.

If a dorsal PIP dislocation is unstable, it will dislocate as the digit is brought into extension. Further treatment varies with the position of redislocation. If closed reduction is easily achieved, the joint is stable in 30° or less of flexion, and the volar avulsion fragment is less than 40% of the articular surface, then extension-block splinting may be used (**Fig. 8**).[17] A dorsal aluminum splint is made to run across the length of the finger with the PIP joint flexed just past the position of stability. The splint is hand-based and uninvolved digits are left free. Full active flexion is allowed immediately. The amount of PIP flexion in the splint is reduced every week by 25% with full extension being achieved at 4 to 6 weeks. Maintenance of reduction must be confirmed by weekly radiographic evaluation. Once full stable extension is obtained, athletes may return to sport with buddy taping used for an additional 3 weeks.

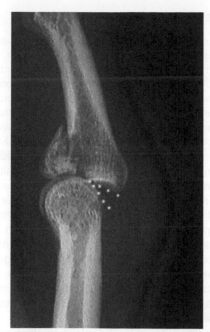

Fig. 7. Radiograph demonstrating the "V" sign (*dotted lines*) that signifies incomplete PIP joint reduction.

Lateral Proximal Interphalangeal Dislocations

Closed reduction is usually successful in restoring joint congruency. Lateral PIP dislocations are reduced under digital block through gentle longitudinal traction followed by radial or ulnar-directed force, depending on the direction of dislocation (ulnar-directed force for radial dislocation and vice versa). Stability is assessed after closed reduction, and if stable, the digit is mobilized with buddy taping to the digit that is adjacent to the injured collateral ligament. Early motion is initiated within buddy taping and can be continued for 3 weeks. Ice and compression are used intermittently to minimize swelling and facilitate movement.

Surgical repair of the torn collateral ligament does ensure joint stability and must be considered in an athlete.[18–22] Indications for surgical repair include postreduction lateral instability of more than 20° on stress testing, involvement of the index or small finger, or high demands placed on the finger by the athlete (eg, baseball pitcher).

Volar Proximal Interphalangeal Dislocations

Volar PIP dislocations are reduced under digital block through gentle longitudinal traction followed by extension at the PIP joint. These injuries usually reduce easily, but must be immobilized in full extension for 3 to 4 weeks to allow the central slip to heal. The DIP is left free and movement is encouraged. DIP motion promotes gliding of the terminal slip, takes tension off the injured central slip, and helps to prevent volar subluxation of the lateral bands. The initial immobilization is followed by dynamic extension splinting that permits active flexion for an additional 2 weeks; this is then followed by passive flexion and strengthening. Irreducible volar PIP dislocations require operative reduction and are likely due to volar-rotatory dislocations with extensor mechanism interposition.

PERCUTANEOUS MANAGEMENT

Percutaneous pinning is an excellent treatment alternative for reducible but unstable PIP dislocations. The pin may be inserted as a blocking pin to prevent full extension, or passed across the joint to immobilize it while soft tissue healing occurs. A blocking wire functions in a similar way to a dorsal extension-blocking splint.[23] The PIP is reduced with axial traction and flexed maximally. A 0.9-mm smooth K-wire is placed percutaneously through the center of the proximal phalanx articular surface. The K-wire is driven retrograde into the proximal phalanx at a 30° angle to its long

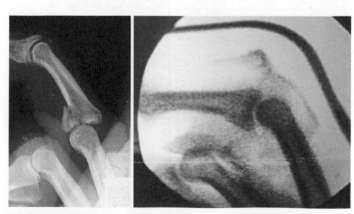

Fig. 8. Treatment of a PIP fracture-dislocation (*left*) with an extension-block splint (*right*).

axis until it engages the volar cortex. The K-wire is bent and left outside the skin and acts as a block to the last 30° of extension (**Fig. 9**). A protective splint is used and gentle active ROM is begun the day after surgery (**Fig. 10**). The K-wire is removed after 3 weeks at which time active and passive ROM are started to regain the remaining PIP extension. In cases of fracture-dislocations, the volar fragment may not be reduced anatomically by this technique; this is not critical as long as the joint is concentrically reduced. Athletes may return to sport after the pin is removed, but should buddy tape the digit until full ROM is achieved and they are asymptomatic.

Another option for unstable injuries is the placement of a transarticular pin after joint reduction. This technique can be applied to dislocations in all directions and does not require any patient compliance. The technique has been applied to unstable dorsal PIP fracture-dislocations involving up to 50% of the articular surface.[24] The PIP joint is reduced and stabilized in 20° to 40° of flexion. A smooth 0.9-mm K-wire is placed in retrograde fashion from the bare area on the dorsum of the middle phalanx, across the PIP joint, and into the head of the proximal phalanx. The pin is left in place for 3 to 4 weeks and an extension-block splint may be used for an additional 2 weeks after pin removal. The athlete should avoid sport during this time. After pin removal, active and passive ROM are initiated and the athlete may return to sport with buddy taping, which should be used until full ROM is achieved and he or she is asymptomatic. Although it may intuitively be expected to cause significant stiffness, the reported results in the setting of dorsal PIP fracture-dislocation are comparable to ORIF.[24,25]

SKELETAL TRACTION

For unstable PIP fracture-dislocations, various methods of skeletal traction, distraction, and dynamic external fixation have been used for treatment.[26–32] These methods are based on the concept of stabilizing the PIP joint and improving fracture alignment by distracting the soft tissues around the base of the middle phalanx, allowing reduction through ligamentotaxis. Use of skeletal traction is appropriate when the PIP joint reduces congruently and the middle phalanx cup-shape is restored. These treatment methods have shown good results in terms of postoperative ROM, return to activity, and patient satisfaction. The technique is especially useful in pilon fractures with fragments too small for internal fixation; the results are comparable to ORIF.[33] The advantages of this technique are avoidance of soft tissue stripping or dissection, early ROM, prevention of soft tissue contractures, and decreased postoperative swelling.

The disadvantages of skeletal traction include the need for pin care, risk of pin track infections, and residual articular incongruity, as skeletal traction does not elevate all depressed and impacted fragments. Reports on posttraumatic arthritis after the use of skeletal fixation have varied results, ranging from 0% to 30%.[29,30] Whereas articular reduction is a secondary goal to joint stabilization and early ROM, joint stability depends on restoration of the middle phalanx volar buttress. In addition, asymmetric fracture fragment depression can lead to unacceptable angulation. In cases that demonstrate asymmetric depression or loss of the middle phalanx cup-shape, additional intervention is required. Reduction can be

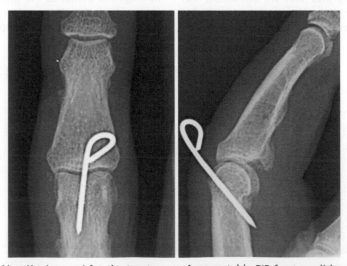

Fig. 9. Extension-blocking K-wire used for the treatment of an unstable PIP fracture-dislocation.

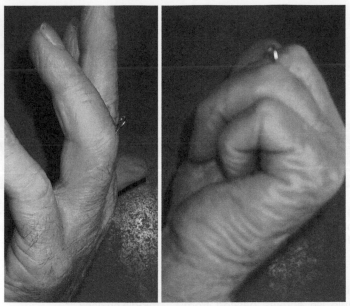

Fig. 10. Hand of a patient with an extension-blocking wire placed for a PIP fracture-dislocation. The patient is encouraged to move the joint through the permitted ROM.

accomplished through percutaneous elevation of impacted fragments with a K-wire or a freer dissector. If these problems cannot be corrected or the joint does not congruently reduce, formal ORIF should be considered.

A simple and economical method of traction uses K-wires to create a low-profile frame.[26] A small, 1.2-mm smooth K-wire is placed transversely across the proximal phalanx condyles, close to the axis of PIP motion. A second K-wire is placed transversely across the distal shaft of the middle phalanx, distal to the fracture. The distal wire is first bent 90° proximally, and this is followed by an S-shaped bend into the wire that allows it to loop around the proximal transverse wire. The configuration generates tension and distracts the PIP joint. Early active motion is allowed and the wires are removed at 3 weeks. Buddy taping should be used until full ROM is achieved and the athlete is asymptomatic. Radiographic widening of the middle phalanx base does occur but has little clinical significance.

OPEN REDUCTION INTERNAL FIXATION

ORIF has a limited but important role in the treatment of unstable dorsal PIP fracture-dislocations. Open reduction is not widely used due to the risk of stiffness, the generally good results of closed and percutaneous treatment, and unstable fracture patterns generally having small, comminuted fracture fragments that are too small for screw

fixation. The indications for ORIF include displacement of a large volar fragment from the middle phalanx that does not reduce, failure to reduce the joint by previous treatments, and cases of late presentation. ORIF has the advantage of restoration of immediate stability that allows early protected ROM with the potential for good to excellent results in selected cases.

Dorsal, volar, and midlateral approaches have been described for dorsal PIP fracture-dislocations.[34–37] The volar approach allows direct visualization of the fracture fragment and permits lag screw fixation and restoration of the volar buttress of the middle phalanx. This procedure uses a volar Bruner approach that extends from the proximal digital crease to the DIP joint crease (**Fig. 11**). The digital neurovascular bundles are mobilized from the flexor sheath. The flexor tendon sheath is opened like a trapdoor between the A2 and A4 pulleys and is reflected laterally. The flexor tendons are retracted to one side to expose the damaged volar plate, which is mobilized by releasing its lateral attachments to the collateral ligaments, and the plate is then reflected proximally. The collateral ligament attachments to the middle phalanx are partially released in a volar to dorsal direction, which allows the digit to be gently hyperextended until it is fully doubled over like a shotgun, exposing the volar fracture.

Small comminuted fracture fragments are removed and the major volar fragment is elevated and reduced provisionally with K-wires. The

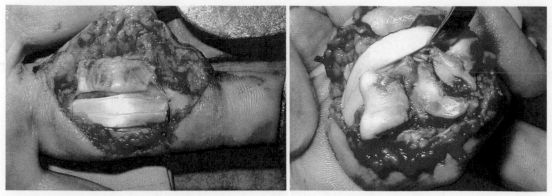

Fig. 11. Intraoperative photos of the volar "shotgun" approach to the PIP joint. The photo on the left demonstrates reflection of the flexor sheath between A2 and A4 pulleys. The final appearance is shown on the right, after the joint is mobilized and dislocated dorsally to allow the middle phalanx to lie parallel to the proximal one. The volar bone fragment can now be fixed easily.

fracture is temporarily stabilized with K-wires that are replaced with two lag screws passed from volar to dorsal (**Fig. 12**). In fractures that are too small or comminuted for screws, one can consider fixation with a circumferential wire loop.[38] Alternatively in small, comminuted fractures, an osteochondral graft from the dorsal lip of the hamate

can be used to reconstruct the volar lip of the middle phalanx.[39]

ORIF is also useful as an adjunct to external fixation or as the primary treatment for pilon fractures of the middle phalanx.[40] Considerable care must be taken to avoid soft tissue stripping and devascularization of the fracture fragments. These

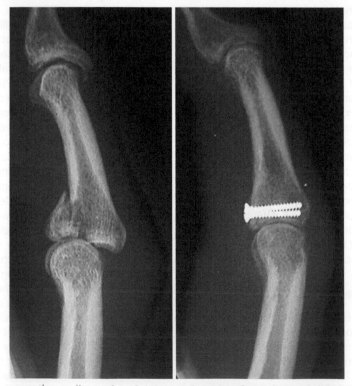

Fig. 12. Pre- and postoperative radiographs of internal fixation of PIP fracture-dislocation using the volar approach.

fractures are best treated through a midlateral approach using an incision defined by the line joining points formed by the flexion creases of the interphalangeal joints when the digit is fully flexed. The dorsal skin flap is elevated, exposing the extensor mechanism lateral band, which is retracted dorsally after dividing the transverse retinacular ligament. The collateral ligament is identified and a longitudinal capsulotomy is made just dorsal to it. Provisional reduction may require K-wires. Definitive fixation is then performed with the use of lag screws directed laterally or from dorsal to volar as needed. The bare area between the lateral bands distal to the central slip insertion is a good location for screw insertion (**Fig. 13**).

Volar PIP dislocations with dorsal lip fractures that are displaced greater than 2 mm or are irreducible require operative fixation. Anatomic reduction of the dorsal lip ensures secure healing of the central slip and restoration of the extensor mechanism. The dorsal fragment can be stabilized with percutaneous or open reduction and lag screw fixation from the dorsal to volar direction.[41] If open reduction is necessary, a curved dorsal skin incision is made over the PIP joint. The extensor mechanism is usually disrupted at the central slip, but additional exposure to reduce the fragment can be gained by making an incision between the lateral band and the extensor slip on one side. The joint is

reduced and may be held with a temporary K-wire. Provisional reduction of the fragment is achieved with a small smooth K-wire, and one or two lag screws are placed dorsal to volar. In comminuted fractures, tension band fixation may be employed instead of screw fixation. Based on the size and stability of fixation, the transarticular pin may be removed after fixation or left in place for 2 weeks, at which time an external splint can be applied. The longitudinal incision in the extensor mechanism is repaired with a running nonabsorbable suture.

The joint is protected postoperatively in full extension with a splint. Protected motion is started around 1 to 2 weeks postoperatively using a Capener splint that provides passive extension of the PIP joint.[34] Protection of the PIP joint in full extension with a small volar splint must be maintained for 6 weeks. The athlete can return to sport as soon as 3 weeks after surgery with splint immobilization of the PIP joint.

RESULTS AND COMPLICATIONS

Stable joint reduction and early ROM positively influence outcomes for PIP fractures and fracture-dislocations. With simple dislocations, most athletes can expect to regain full flexion; however, a small flexion contracture is common and, fortunately, rarely symptomatic. With fracture-

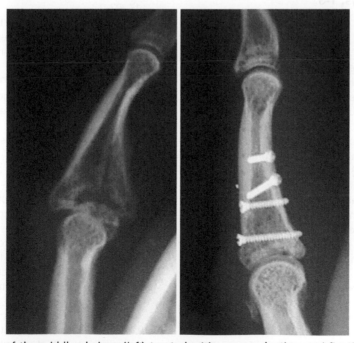

Fig. 13. Pilon fracture of the middle phalanx (*left*) treated with open reduction and fixation with multiple lag screws using a lateral approach (*right*).

dislocations, long-term studies have shown radiographic degenerative changes in as many as 96% of patients treated with ORIF; however, the majority report little or no pain, do not have difficulty with work activities, and do not need modifications in their leisure activities.[42] The usual ROM averages from 12° of extension to 80° of flexion. Delaying ORIF of unstable PIP fracture-dislocations, and thereby delaying rehabilitation and ROM exercises, has been associated with decreased postoperative ROM.[38]

The results of ORIF are comparable to those of percutaneous pinning, which shows 90% good functional recovery and an average PIP ROM of 85° with an average flexion contracture of 8°.[25] The average PIP ROM after external fixation of PIP fracture-dislocations has been reported to be similar, between 74° and 88°.[26–29,31] Complications of ORIF include dislocation, reported in up to 11% of patients. Redislocations involve loss of fixation and are associated with a poor outcome; up to 67% of these patients require either arthroplasty or arthrodesis. Deep infection and stiffness requiring tenolysis are more common after surgical treatment and have been reported in up to 4% of patients.

ACKNOWLEDGMENTS

The authors acknowledge and thank Patrick Carrico, MAMS, who prepared the diagrammatic pictures used in **Figs. 1–3**.

REFERENCES

1. Leibovic SJ, Bowers WH. Anatomy of the proximal interphalangeal joint. Hand Clin 1994;10:169–78.
2. Kuczynski K. The proximal interphalangeal joint: anatomy and causes of stiffness in the fingers. J Bone Joint Surg Br 1968;50(3):656–63.
3. Minamikawa Y, Horri E, Amadio PC, et al. Stability and constraint of the proximal interphalangeal joint. J Hand Surg [Am] 1993;18:198–204.
4. Bindra R. Dislocations and fracture dislocations of the metacarpophalangeal and proximal interphalangeal joints. In: Ring DC, Cohen MS, editors. Fractures of the hand and wrist. New York: Informa Healthcare; 2007. p. 41–74.
5. Glickel SZ, Barron OA, Eaton RG. Dislocations and ligament injuries in the digits. In: Green DP, Hotchkiss RN, Pederson WC, editors. 4th edition, Green's operative hand surgery, vol. 1. New York: Churchill Livingstone; 1999. p. 772–808.
6. Bowers WH, Wolf JW Jr, Nehil JL, et al. The proximal interphalangeal joint. J Hand Surg [Am] 1980;5: 79–88.
7. Kraemer BA, Gilula LA. Phalangeal fractures and dislocations. In: Gilula LA, editor. The traumatized hand and wrist. Philadelphia: W.B. Sanders; 1992. p. 105–70.
8. Blazar PE, Steinberg DR. Fractures of the proximal interphalangeal joint. J Am Acad Orthop Surg 2000;8:383–90.
9. Kiefhaber TR, Stern PJ. Clinical perspective: fracture dislocations of the proximal interphalangeal joint. J Hand Surg [Am] 1998;23:369–80.
10. Spinner M, Choi BY. Anterior dislocation of the proximal interphalangeal joint: a cause of rupture of the central slip of the extensor mechanism. J Bone Joint Surg Am 1970;52:1329–36.
11. Inoue G, Maeda N. Irreducible palmar dislocation of the proximal interphalangeal joint of the finger. J Hand Surg [Am] 1990;15:301–4.
12. Boden RA, Srinivasan MS. Rotational dislocation of the proximal interphalangeal joint of the finger. J Bone Joint Surg Br 2008;90(3):385–6.
13. Akagi T, Hashizume H, Inoue H, et al. Computer simulation analysis of fracture dislocation of the proximal interphalangeal joint using the finite element method. Acta Med Okayama 1994;48:263–70.
14. Schenck R. Classification of fractures and dislocations of the proximal interphalangeal joint. Hand Clin 1994;10:179–85.
15. Light TR. Buttress pinning techniques. Orthop Rev 1981;10:49–55.
16. Lutz M, Fritz D, Arora R, et al. Anatomical basis for functional treatment of dorsolateral dislocation of the proximal interphalangeal joint. Clin Anat 2004; 17:303–7.
17. McElfresh EC, Dobyns JH, O'Brien ET. Management of the proximal interphalangeal joints by extension-block splinting. J Bone Joint Surg Am 1972;54: 1705–10.
18. Redler I, Williams JT. Rupture of a collateral ligament of the proximal interphalangeal joint of the finger: analysis of 18 cases. J Bone Joint Surg Am 1967; 49:322–6.
19. McCue FC, Honner R, Johnson MC, et al. Athletic injuries of the proximal interphalangeal joint requiring surgical treatment. J Bone Joint Surg Am 1970;52:937–56.
20. Ali MS. Complete disruption of collateral mechanism of proximal interphalangeal joint of fingers. J Hand Surg [Br] 1984;9B:191–3.
21. Isani A, Melone CP. Ligamentous injuries of the hand in athletes. Clin Sports Med 1986;5:757–72.
22. Brunet ME, Haddad RJ. Fractures and dislocations of the metacarpals and phalanges. Clin Sports Med 1986;5:773–81.
23. Viegas SF. Extension block pinning for proximal phalanx interphalangeal joint fracture dislocations: preliminary report of a new technique. J Hand Surg [Am] 1992;17:896–901.

24. Newington DP, Davis TR, Barton NJ. The treatment of dorsal fracture-dislocation of the proximal interphalangeal joint by closed reduction and Kirschner wire fixation: a 16-year follow up. J Hand Surg [Br] 2001;26:537–40.

25. Aladin A, Davis TR. Dorsal fracture-dislocation of the proximal interphalangeal joint: a comparative study of percutaneous Kirschner wire fixation versus open reduction and internal fixation. J Hand Surg [Br] 2005;30:120–8.

26. Hynes MC, Giddins GE. Dynamic external fixation for pilon fractures of the interphalangeal joints. J Hand Surg [Br] 2001;26:122–4.

27. Majumder S, Peck F, Watson JS, et al. Lessons learned from the management of complex intra-articular fractures at the base of the middle phalanges of fingers. J Hand Surg [Br] 2003;28:559–65.

28. Ellis SJ, Cheng R, Prokopis P, et al. Treatment of proximal interphalangeal dorsal fracture-dislocation injuries with dynamic external fixation: a pins and rubber band system. J Hand Surg [Am] 2007;32:1242–50.

29. Ruland RT, Hogan CJ, Cannon DL, et al. Use of dynamic distraction external fixation for unstable fracture-dislocations of the proximal interphalangeal joint. J Hand Surg [Am] 2008;33:19–25.

30. Agee JM. Unstable fracture dislocations of the proximal interphalangeal joint: treatment with the force couple splint. Clin Orthop 1987;214:101–12.

31. Krakauer JD, Stern PJ. Hinged device for fractures involving the proximal interphalangeal joint. Clin Orthop 1996;327:29–37.

32. Johnson D, Tiernan E, Richards AM, et al. Dynamic external fixation for complex intraarticular phalangeal fractures. J Hand Surg [Br] 2004;29:76–81.

33. Stern PJ, Roman RJ, Kiefhaber TR. Pilon fractures of the proximal interphalangeal joint. J Hand Surg [Am] 1991;16:844–50.

34. Hamilton SC, Stern PJ, Fassler PR, et al. Mini-screw fixation for the treatment of proximal interphalangeal joint dorsal fracture-dislocations. J Hand Surg [Am] 2006;31:1349–54.

35. Lee JY, Teoh LC. Dorsal fracture dislocations of the proximal interphalangeal joint treated by open reduction and interfragmentary screw fixation: indications, approaches, and results. J Hand Surg [Br] 2006;31:138–46.

36. Wilson JN, Rowland SA. Fracture-dislocation of the proximal interphalangeal joint of the finger: treatment by open reduction and internal fixation. J Bone Joint Surg Am 1966;48:493–502.

37. Grant I, Berger AC, Tham SK. Internal fixation of unstable fracture dislocations of the proximal interphalangeal joint. J Hand Surg [Br] 2005;30: 492–8.

38. Weiss AP. Cerclage fixation for fracture dislocation of the proximal interphalangeal joint. Clin Orthop 1996;327:21–8.

39. Williams RM, Kiefhaber TR, Sommerkamp TG, et al. Treatment of unstable dorsal proximal interphalangeal fracture/dislocations using a hemi-hamate autograft. J Hand Surg [Am] 2003;28: 856–65.

40. Sarris I, Goitz RJ, Sotereanos DG. Dynamic traction and minimal internal fixation for thumb and digital pilon fractures. J Hand Surg [Am] 2004; 29:39–43.

41. Tekkis PP, Kessaris N, Gavalas M, et al. The role of mini-fragment screw fixation in volar dislocations of the proximal interphalangeal joint. Arch Orthop Trauma Surg 2001;121:121–2.

42. Deitch MA, Kiefhaber TR, Comisar BR, et al. Dorsal fracture dislocations of the proximal interphalangeal joint: surgical complications and long-term results. J Hand Surg [Am] 1999;24:914–23.

Acute Ulnar Collateral Ligament Injury in the Athlete

Jeff W. Johnson, MD[a,b,c], Randall W. Culp, MD, FACS[a,d],*

KEYWORDS

- Ulnar collateral ligament • Gamekeeper's • Skier's
- CMC arthroscopy • Thumb metacarpophalangeal joint

The functional thumb is a necessity for successful athletic participation. It not only allows the athlete to manipulate athletic equipment but also allows the precise manipulation of objects in the athlete's hand. Injury to the thumb often negates power grip and finesse of the athletic hand. Injuries can range from fractures, to dislocations, to ligamentous injuries. The relatively unconstrained thumb metacarpophalangeal (MP) joint is particularly vulnerable to injury from an abduction moment to its distal segment. Such injuries occur both from direct contact and with falls on equipment such as racquet handles and ski poles. The stability of the athlete's MP joint must be restored to allow for a productive return to sport.

ANATOMY

The MP joint of the thumb allows for motion in multiple planes simultaneously. The major arc of motion is flexion and extension; however, a small amount of abduction and adduction is possible. Since the lateral condyle of the metacarpal head has a larger radius of curvature than the medial condyle, the distal motion segment undergoes slight pronation as flexion increases. The metacarpal head radius of curvature is quite variable, with flat heads having less motion than those with a more spherical shape. There is little inherent stability from the articulation of the proximal

phalanx with the metacarpal head. Capsular and ligamentous structures restrain the articulation during loaded activities. Collateral ligaments are divided into proper and accessory bundles. The proper ligaments originate from the lateral condyle of the metacarpal head 3 mm from its dorsal surface and 7 mm from the joint, pass obliquely across the MP joint to insert in the volar half of the proximal phalanx base approximately 8 mm from the dorsal surface and 3 mm from the joint.[1] The accessory ligaments are more volar with respect to the proper bundle, inserting onto the volar plate (**Fig. 1**). The proper bundle is tight in flexion and loose in extension, with the accessory bundle tight in extension and loose in flexion. The volar aspect of the MP joint is supported by the volar plate; however, in the thumb this structure does not possess checkrein ligaments. The adductor pollicis inserts into the ulnar sesamoid whereas the flexor pollicis brevis and abductor pollicis insert into the radial sesamoid, both providing some dynamic stability to the articulation. These muscles also attach to the extensor mechanism, thereby providing dynamic lateral support.[2]

INJURY PATTERNS

Although injury may occur to either the radial collateral ligament (RCL) or the ulnar collateral

[a] Philadelphia Hand Center, 700 South Henderson Road, Suite 200, King of Prussia, PA 19406, USA
[b] Department of Orthopaedic Surgery, University of Arkansas for Medical Sciences, 4301 West Markham Street, Slot 531, Little Rock, AR 72205, USA
[c] 925 Chestnut Street, Philadelphia, PA 19106, USA
[d] Department of Orthopaedic, Hand and Microsurgery, Thomas Jefferson University, Philadelphia, PA, USA
* Corresponding author. Department of Orthopaedic, Hand and Microsurgery, Thomas Jefferson University, Philadelphia, PA.
E-mail address: rwculp@handcenters.com (R. Culp).

Hand Clin 25 (2009) 437–442
doi:10.1016/j.hcl.2009.05.014
0749-0712/09/$ – see front matter © 2009 Elsevier Inc. All rights reserved.

hand.theclinics.com

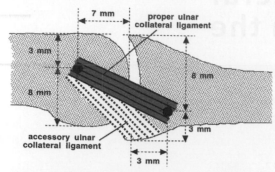

Fig. 1. Anatomic attachment of ulnar collateral ligaments of the thumb. (*From* Bean HG, Tencer AF, Trumble TE. The effect of thumb metacarpophalangeal ulnar collateral ligament attachment site on joint range of motion: an in vitro study. J Hand Surg Am 1999;24(2):283–7; with permission.)

ligament (UCL), injury to the latter has been noted to be 10 times more common.[2] Injury to the UCL is often the result of rapid abduction of the thumb. This may occur as the result of force applied directly to the thumb or in the instance of a fall on an outstretched hand with an abducted thumb. The eponym associated with this injury, "skier's thumb," was coined after UCL injury was observed in skiers falling with a ski pole handle in hand, causing an abduction moment to the thumb.[3] Although not limited to skiing injuries, increased incidence has been noted on the artificial plastic ski mats often used in Europe and Japan.[4] Not only does this mechanism injure the UCL, but it may be associated with damage to the dorsal capsule and the ulnar aspect of the volar plate. The UCL is five times more likely to tear at its distal insertion, although proximal and mid substance tears do occur.

Volar subluxation of the proximal phalanx in relation to the metacarpal head is thought to be related to concomitant tears of the UCL and the stabilizing dorsal capsule. The intact RCL acts as a pivot, around which the distal segment rotates into supination, thus giving rise to subluxation of the MP joint. The abductor pollicis brevis causes a radial shift of the proximal phalanx; however, the adductor pollicis does not affect MP joint motion.[5] Fractures may also occur, most commonly of the ulnar aspect of the proximal phalangeal base. Fracture fragments are generally small, but may be large enough to necessitate reduction, especially if displaced more than 2 mm.[6] Care should be taken to evaluate for associated fractures, such as shearing patterns of the proximal phalanx base or of the metacarpal head. Salter-Harris fractures are possible, but less common. Associated fractures include

Bennett fractures, which may mask an associated injury to the collateral mechanism.[7]

Perhaps the most well recognized pattern of injury to the UCL is seen in cases where the ligament is completely torn from its distal insertion. The ligament may displace as the distal segment of the thumb continues to abduct from the initial deforming force, pulling the UCL from underneath the aponeurosis of the adductor pollicis. The UCL then becomes trapped outside the aponeurosis, and is unlikely to heal in this position. The stump of the torn UCL is often palpable in this superficial position. This injury was originally described in 1962 by Stener and thus bears his name in its common terminology, "the Stener lesion" (**Fig. 2**).[8] The completely displaced segment of the UCL is seen in 64% to 87% of injuries, according to some sources.[8,9]

DIAGNOSIS

Athletes often present with ecchymosis, swelling, and pain along the ulnar border of the thumb. History is important, as the mechanism may give clues as to the nature of the injury. If injury to the UCL is suspected, radiographs should be obtained before stress testing the joint, as this may shift a nondisplaced fracture. Stability of the joint should be assessed by stabilizing the metacarpal and placing an abduction moment on the distal segment of the thumb. Although several

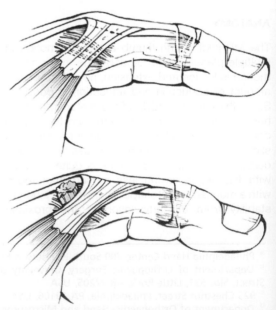

Fig. 2. Stener lesion. (*From* Bucholz RW, Heckman JD. Fractures and dislocations in the hand. In: Rockwood and Green's fractures in adults. 5th edition. Philadelphia: Lippincott Williams & Wilkins; 2001. p. 819; with permission.)

authors have suggested values for establishing the existence of injury, generally 30° of laxity both in extension and at 30° of MP flexion or greater than 15° difference from the contralateral joint indicates a UCL tear.[10,11] In cases where instability is noted in flexion alone (extension is stable), it is believed that the accessory UCL is intact.[10] However, instability in extension alone may indicate a volar plate injury.[12] Complete tears may be distinguished from a Grade 2 sprain by the presence of definite endpoint during stress to an incompletely torn UCL. Local anesthetic has been shown to be helpful in the identification of tears when pain precludes examination.[13]

As mentioned before, radiography is a necessary adjunct in the evaluation of injury to the UCL. In addition to three standard radiographic views, some clinicians advocate the use of stress views, although this carries with it a risk for fragment displacement. Static x-rays may also provide information if volar subluxation of the proximal phalanx is seen. This "Sag Sign" indicates the loss of the ulnar stabilizing structures, allowing the proximal phalanx to supinate with respect to the metacarpal head.[14] Standard arthrograms may be useful, but are not routinely done. A positive arthrogram shows contrast extravasation into the footprint of the ligament attachment or contrast escape by way of a capsular tear; however, the latter is not purely indicative of

a UCL tear. Several studies have evaluated the utility of MRI or ultrasound to discern the extent of UCL injury. Ultrasound is quite accurate and readily available in most centers, but it requires some expertise to identify the anatomic structures of interest. MRI was also found to be useful, but its resolution is often limited by the MRI equipment. Dedicated extremity (wrist or digit) coils were shown to provide adequate resolution to identify tears. Some advocate the use of intra-articular gadolinium to enhance the ability to detect a Stener lesion, although this comes at some expense. Accurate identification has been shown with today's high-resolution scanners (at least 1.5 T) and dedicated extremity coils.[15]

TREATMENT

Incomplete injuries of the UCL may be treated with immobilization, either with a thermoplastic thumb spica or, in cases where early return to play is required, a thumb spica cast, leaving the interphalangeal (IP) joint of the thumb free. One should be familiar with the local sporting regulations when choosing the style of immobilization, as the rules often vary between regions. Full-time immobilization should continue for a period of approximately 4 weeks, followed by an additional period of 2 to 4 weeks of immobilization during play, when active range of motion exercises begin off the field.

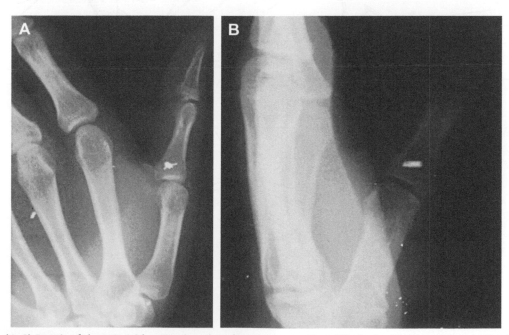

Fig. 3. (*A, B*) Repair of the UCL with a Mitek anchor. (*From* Beauperthuy GD, Burke EF. Alternative method of repairing collateral ligament injuries at the metacarpophalangeal joints of the thumb and fingers. J Hand Surg Br 1997;22(6):736–8; with permission.)

Immobilization in the case of complete UCL rupture has not been consistently successful, and thus surgical repair is recommended to allow return to competitive play.[16]

Operative treatment of UCL injuries varies depending on the nature of the rupture. The most common scenario is that of a distal avulsion from the base of the proximal phalanx. Ryu and Fagan[17]

advocated arthroscopic reduction of the UCL without fixation of the torn ligament. Once the insertion site was debrided with the aid of the scope, the UCL was returned to its anatomic position and the thumb was held in 20° to 30° of flexion for approximately 4 weeks, after which functional bracing began. This technique may be used in the case of displaced ligamentous injuries with

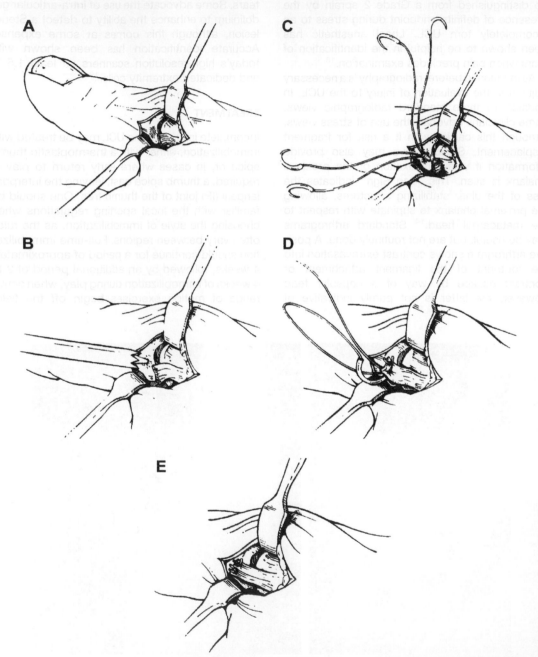

Fig. 4. (A–E) Technique for placement of Mitek anchor. (From Weiland AJ, Berner SH, Hotchkiss RN, et al. Repair of acute ulnar collateral ligament injuries of the thumb metacarpophalangeal joint with an intraosseous suture anchor. J Hand Surg Am 1997;22:585–91; with permission.)

adductor interposition. Other authors have used arthroscopy as an adjunct for fixation of the ligament to its anatomic insertion. Suture anchors may be used to reestablish the distal anchor point, once reduction is achieved arthroscopically. It is the authors' experience that open reduction and fixation of the completely ruptured UCL performs similarly to the aforementioned techniques. Open treatment has the additional benefit of providing excellent exposure should fracture fixation be required for avulsions of the proximal phalangeal base.[11]

Open treatment begins with a dorsoulnar incision centered over the MP joint of the thumb. Care should be taken to identify and gently retract the dorsal sensory branches of the radial nerve, as these structures are easily irritated, which causes postoperative paresthesias. Identifying the adductor pollicis aponeurosis and opening the proximal four-fifths exposes the underlying capsule of the MP joint of the thumb. This structure is then opened longitudinally, taking care to develop and protect this structure for later repair. The UCL lies just beneath the capsule along the ulnar border of the metacarpal head. Any amorphous scar that may have developed since the injury should be removed, to allow for direct ligament apposition to bone. At this point the insertion site for the ligament is prepared by removing the periosteum from the ulnar base of the proximal phalanx. The surface of the bone is denuded using a small curette. The MP joint is then pinned in a slightly overcorrected (ulnar deviated) position using a 0.045″ Kirschner wire. The pin is left out of the skin (dorsal-lateral aspect of proximal phalanx) to allow the surgeon to remove it in the office. A mini suture anchor with 2-0 nonabsorbable suture (Mini-Mitek) is used for the repair, and care should be taken by the surgeon to direct the prongs of the anchor away from the articular surface of the proximal phalangeal base. The anchor is placed just below the midline on the base of the proximal phalanx to recreate the normal anatomic attachment site for the UCL. Careful attention to anchor placement should be used, as nonanatomic positions may lead to loss of MP flexion or failure to stabilize the MP joint to radially directed forces.[1] Once the anchor is in place the sutures are passed into the ligament and tied (**Figs. 3** and **4**). Some authors advocate a second, free suture passed between the distal end of the ligament and the volar plate to reestablish this preexisting relationship. The capsule is then repaired with an absorbable suture, as is the aponeurosis of the adductor pollicis. If a fracture accompanies the UCL rupture, this fragment is repaired using either a small screw or a pin if

appropriate. Tension band wiring has also been described for this injury.[18] If the fragment is too small for fixation, it is excised and the suture anchor is placed in such a manner as to allow the ligament to be advanced into the bed of the fracture. The skin is closed and a thumb spica splint is applied, leaving the IP joint of the thumb and the MP joints of the remaining digits free. The skin sutures are removed in 7 to 10 days, and active motion is begun for the thumb IP and digits of the hand. The postoperative splint is exchanged for a forearm based thermoplastic thumb spica, again leaving the IP of the thumb free. The pin is removed 4 weeks later, and active motion starts at that time, continuing splint immobilization outside of therapy sessions for a total of 6 to 8 weeks. Early motion is safe as long as strict nonloaded exercises are used, as repair failure occurs at three times the load generated by early motion protocols.[19] Play resumes once the pin is removed and the thumb is in a well padded thermoplastic splint or cast with thumb spica leaving the IP joint free. Unprotected play starts 12 weeks postoperatively while protection of the thumb by taping continues. Patients have shown some loss of motion at the MP joint, but they can be expected to gain 75% of their pre-injury strength after healing is complete.[20]

REFERENCES

1. Bean HG, Tencer AF, Trumble TE. The effect of thumb metacarpophalangeal ulnar collateral ligament attachment site on joint range of motion: an in vitro study. J Hand Surg Am 1999;24(2):283–7.
2. Glickel SZ, Barron OA, Catalano LW. Dislocations and ligaments injuries in the digits. In: Green DP, Hotchkiss RN, Pederson WC, et al, editors. Green's operative hand surgery. 5th edition. Philadelphia: Elsevier; 2005. p. 367–73.
3. Fairhurst M, Hansen L. Treatment of "Gamekeeper's thumb" by reconstruction of the ulnar collateral ligament. J Hand Surg Br 2002;27(6):542–5.
4. Keramidas E, Miller G. Adult hand injuries on artificial ski slopes. Ann Plast Surg 2005;55(4):357–8.
5. Draganich LF, Greenspahn S, Mass DP. Effects of the adductor pollicis and abductor pollicis brevis on thumb metacarpophalangeal joint laxity before and after ulnar collateral ligament reconstruction. J Hand Surg Am 2004;29(3):481–8.
6. Giele H, Martin J. The two-level ulnar collateral ligament injury of the metacarpophalangeal joint of the thumb. J Hand Surg Br 2003;28(1):92–3.
7. Smith I, Jamieson A. A rare combined fracture and ligamentous injury of the thumb. J Hand Surg Br 1998;23(4):542–3.

8. Stener B. Displacement of the ruptured ulnar collateral ligament of the metacarpophalangeal joint of the thumb: a clinical and anatomical study. J Bone Joint Surg Br 1962;44:869–79.

9. Heyman P, Gelberman RH, Duncan K, et al. Injuries of the thumb metacarpophalangeal joint: Biomechanical and prospective clinical studies on the usefulness of valgus stress testing. Clin Orthop 1993;292:165–71.

10. Morgan WJ, Slowman LS. Acute hand and wrist injuries in athletes: evaluation and management. J Am Acad Orthop Surg 2001;9:389–400.

11. Osterman AL, Hayden G, Bora FW Jr. Quantitative evaluation of thumb function after ulnar collateral repair and reconstruction. J Trauma 1981;21:854–61.

12. Lee SJ, Montgomery K. Athletic hand injuries. Orthop Clin North Am 2002;33:547–54.

13. Cooper JG, Johnstone AJ, Hider P, et al. Local anaesthetic infiltration increases the accuracy of assessment of ulnar collateral ligament injuries. Emerg Med Australias 2005;17:132–6.

14. Gurdezi S, Mok D. "Sag sign" – a simple radiological sign for detecting injury to the thumb ulnar collateral ligament. J Injury 2008;39(5):191.

15. Peterson JJ, Bancroft LW, Kransdorf MJ, et al. Evaluation of collateral ligament injuries of the metacarpophalangeal joints with magnetic resonance imaging and magnetic resonance arthrography. Curr Probl Diagn Radiol 2007;36:11–20.

16. Dinowitz M, Trumble T, Hanel D, et al. Failure of cast immobilization for thumb ulnar collateral ligament avulsion fractures. J Hand Surg Am 1997;22:1057–63.

17. Ryu J, Fagan R. Arthroscopic treatment of acute complete thumb metacarpophalangeal ulnar collateral ligament tears. J Hand Surg 1995;20A:1037–42.

18. Jupiter JB, Sheppard JE. Tension wire fixation of avulsion fractures in the hand. Clin Orthop Relat Res 1987;214:113–20.

19. Harley BJ, Werner FW, Green JK. A biomechanical modeling of injury, repair, and rehabilitation of ulnar collateral ligament injuries of the thumb. J Hand Surg Am 2004;29(5):915–20.

20. Beauperthuy GD, Burke EF. Alternative method of repairing collateral ligament injuries at the metacarpophalangeal joints of the thumb and fingers. J Hand Surg Br 1997;22(6):736–8.

Bracing and Rehabilitation for Wrist and Hand Injuries in Collegiate Athletes

Shannon Singletary, DPT, ATC, CSCS[a],*, William B. Geissler, MD[b,c]

KEYWORDS

- Wrist injuries • Hand injuries • Compressive forces
- Rehabilitation • Protective bracing • Strength
- Range of motion • Splints

Athletic trainers, physical therapists, and sports-medicine physicians who care for athletic injuries spend a great deal of time in prevention of and care for hand and wrist injuries (wrist and hand trauma constitute up to 9% of all athletic injuries).[1] A Division 1A collegiate sports program will spend in the range of $25,000 to $40,000 per year on preventive bracing, splinting, and taping products for injuries of the wrist and hand. Acute and chronic injuries and conditions to the wrist may result from compressive forces, excessive range of motion (ROM), and repetitive stresses. Normal ROM and stability of the wrist are required for participation in most athletic activities.[2] Prevention of soft-tissue injuries, such as ligament and tendon injuries, are the most common reasons for the use of preventive bracing and taping, whereas injuries to the bones of the hand and wrist are the most common reason for casting and splinting. When injuries do occur, rehabilitation is used to protect and regain sensation, strength, ROM, and function. This article focuses on preventive bracing, protective padding, and rehabilitation for common wrist and hand injuries.

COMMON INJURIES

Some of the most common injuries of the hand and wrist that are seen in collegiate sports are collateral ligament tears, proximal and distal interphalangeal (IP) joint dislocations, metacarpal fractures, scaphoid fractures, and wrist ligamentous injuries. Hand fractures constitute one-quarter to one-third of all fractures that occur during athletic competition.[3] Eighty five percent of all hand fractures that occur in sports happen while playing American football, basketball, or lacrosse. American football has the highest rate of hand fractures among sports, accounting for 50% of all hand fractures. Two-thirds of all hand fractures are metacarpal fractures.[4] Collateral ligament tears to any of the five digits are particularly common in contact sports. Sports such as football and basketball, in which the use of the hands in tackling or fighting for position on the court, often result in a valgus or varus stress to the proximal interphalangeal (PIP) joint. Sprains or complete tears occur to the ligaments of this joint as forces are applied from pulled jerseys or a lever-type force is applied to the tip of the distal phalanx. Baseball players often suffer from direct lever-type forces while sliding head first into a base, with the fingertips extended. Collateral ligament tears of the fingers are most often referred to by coaches and players as the famous "jammed finger." Common deformities of the distal interphalangeal (PIP) joint occur in sports such as basketball and football as a result

a Department of Athletics, University of Mississippi Medical Center, University of Mississippi, 1810 Manning Way, Jackson, MS 38677, USA
b Division of Hand and Upper Extremity Surgery, University of Mississippi Medical Center, 2500 North State Street, Jackson, MS 39216, USA
c Section of Arthroscopic Surgery and Sports Medicine, Department of Orthopaedic Surgery and Rehabilitation, University of Mississippi Medical Center, 2500 North State Street, Jackson, MS 39216, USA
* Corresponding author.
E-mail address: shannon@olemiss.edu (S. Singletary).

Hand Clin 25 (2009) 443–448
doi:10.1016/j.hcl.2009.05.012
0749-0712/09/$ – see front matter © 2009 Elsevier Inc. All rights reserved.

of the ball striking the tip of the finger and resulting in what is referred to as a mallet finger deformity. The most common dislocations of the hand include the volar and dorsal dislocations of the PIP and DIP joints.

Isolated wrist sprains are not as common; however, athletes do fall on the outstretched arm with the wrist extended greater than 90°. This is the mechanism for scaphoid fractures. Scaphoid fractures to the wrist constitute 60% to 70% of all wrist fractures.[5] When ligamentous injuries occur to the wrist, the scapholunate ligament or the triangular fibrocartilage complex is often affected. These injuries are often prevented with proper bracing and taping. However, when the injuries do occur, management consists of rehabilitation and proper steps for early return to play measures. These steps include proper padding either by bracing, casting, or taping. Finally, rehabilitation is usually a process that continues before returning to play and is continued until the injury has made maximum recovery.

PREVENTION

Although preventing all injuries to the hand and wrist is impossible, experienced sports-medicine personnel do their best to prevent the most common injuries when the athlete's sport position duties allow, such as taping the wrist. Prevention of common athletic wrist injuries is often accomplished by several bracing and taping techniques. Bracing and taping techniques are customized to the athlete's position. The fundamental principle of preventive bracing and taping is to provide support, limit excessive ROM, and allow for protection against forces that cause injury. Supplies that are used include cloth athletic tape, neoprene, and sometimes a thermoplastic material.

The wrist is often taped as a preventive measure in sports such as gymnastics and football. These two sports subject athletes to forceful loading of the wrist in an extended position. For example, offensive linemen in football must extend the wrist while applying a direct force to the body of a defensive player during pass blocking. Gymnasts often must support their body weight. In both sports, there are direct forces to the extended wrist that may result in potential injuries. **Fig. 1** shows the classic taping technique for the wrist. This technique prevents excessive wrist extension and flexion. **Fig. 2** shows an "X" technique that provides extra support to limit the appropriate excessive direction. The "X" is applied to the volar side of the hand and wrist it limiting extension is the desired objective. The "X" is applied to the

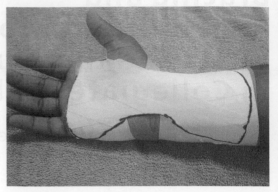

Fig. 1. The "X" technique prevents excessive wrist extension and flexion.

dorsum of the hand and wrist if limiting flexion is the desired objective. There are several keys to remember about this taping technique. First of all, the "X" must be anchored (secured) at both ends of the "X" as shown in the figure. Second, the tape must be long enough so that there is enough of a lever arm on both sides of the joint to actually prevent excessive motion. If the tape does not go far enough distally and proximally, forces applied to the wrist will not be prevented, and the athlete is more likely to injure the wrist. There are also several off-the-shelf prophylactic wrist braces that can be used to limit wrist hyperextension primarily. Although the athlete perceives prophylactic bracing as cumbersome, these braces are usually cost-efficient. By limiting hyperextension of the wrist, injuries such as scapholunate ligament tears and scaphoid fractures can be prevented.

In sports such as basketball and football, the IP joint of the thumb is also taped for injury prevention. **Fig. 3** shows how the collateral ligaments of the thumb are supported. Again, the tape is applied so that there is an opposite preventive force applied when a direct varus or valgus force is applied in the opposite direction. There has

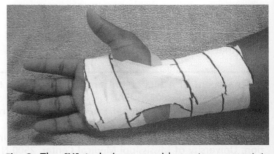

Fig. 2. The "X" technique provides extra support to limit the appropriate excessive direction. The "X" supplies the volar side of the hand and wrist if limiting extension is the desired objective.

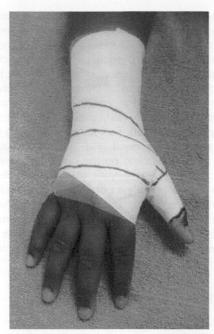

Fig. 3. The tape is applied so that the opposite preventive force resists direct varus or valgus force when applied in the opposite direction. This taping technique supports the collateral ligaments of the thumb.

been a long-standing argument among experts as to whether cloth tape applies enough force to actually prevent injury. Research has shown that cloth athletic tape loosens up soon with athletic activity and, therefore, cannot prevent injury. However, other research has shown that applying cloth tape to joints of the body, such as the wrist, knee, ankle, or even shoulder, actually improves proprioception (kinesthetic awareness) and thus increases dynamic stability of the joint.

REHABILITATION

Rehabilitation of hand and wrist injuries in sports requires teamwork between the physician, athlete, therapist, and/or athletic trainer. The stages of rehabilitation include initial tissue healing, recovery of motion and flexibility, recovery of strength and power, recovery of endurance, and return to routine activities on the playing field.[6]

Recovery of motion is the most important aspect of rehabilitation. It has been well documented that a few millimeters of motion prevents debilitating adhesions. The inexperienced athletic trainer or physical therapist will concentrate too early on strengthening because the patient is an athlete. Too often, basic ROM exercises are believed to be too conservative and not sport-specific. Inexperienced coaches have contributed to this noncompliance by generalizing all finger

injuries as being a "jammed finger." In such cases, the standard treatment protocol has always been buddy taping the injured finger to the finger next to it and returning to play. Physicians and therapists often see athletes who have been given this treatment after the season, and the athletes have adhesions and nonfunctional ROM. The athlete is left trying to compete in a sport with a grip strength that is fair at best. For the multisport high school athlete, this means that after football season, the athlete is unable to grip a bat or stick to begin preparing for the next sport. However, gaining acceptable ROM is essential before functional strength gains can be achieved (specific exercises to gain ROM). To regain full ROM in the injured fingers, edema must be controlled. If left alone, fluid within the joints forms fibrous scar tissue that blocks the normal mechanics of the finger joints. Therapists and athletic trainers must keep in mind two kinematic characteristics of the fingers, with the exception of the thumb. First, the four metacarpophalangeal (MP) joints are condyloid with only 2° of freedom. Second, IP joints (proximal and distal) have 1° of freedom. The primary motions of both joints are flexion and extension.[7] Swelling that is not addressed easily blocks the primary movement that allows for gripping motions. Control or decrease of swelling to the fingers may be achieved by retrograde massage, proper elevation, compression, and icing immediately after therapy or participation in sports. Early emphasis on controlling edema is paramount to a successful return to play. Retrograde massage should be performed by the rehabilitation professional by placing the athlete's fingers in an elevated position (above the heart), gripping the athlete's swollen digit distally, and sliding the therapist's fingers in a proximal direction to the head of the metacarpals. This gives the therapist a vision of a wave-like action to the edema. Hand or massage lotion can be used to decrease friction and allow for an easy glide. This can easily be taught to the athlete so that the athlete can perform the maneuver frequently throughout the day. Surgically repaired fingers, with healing incisions or open wounds, require care to work around the incision. Other tips to control swelling in the athlete's hand would be to wear compressive gloves while he or she is not in therapy. The injured athlete should keep the hand elevated above the heart while not in therapy, to minimize swelling. Holding the injured hand in the dependent position quickly causes swelling to pool within the involved digit. Finally, when appropriate, performing active/passive ROM to the digit with hand placed in an elevated position decreases swelling and reduces the likelihood of the nonfunctional stiff joint. Synchronous wrist and digital tenodesis exercises and individual joint-blocking exercises are two excellent nonresistive exercises to begin early to regain maximum ROM in all digital joints.

Joint-blocking exercises are used in collateral ligament tears, phalangeal fractures, and, when appropriate, flexor tendon repairs. The experienced therapist and athletic trainer recognize that the wrist plays a vital role in rehabilitation of the fingers. Many times, injured patients drop their wrists into slight flexion, even while pain is controlled in the fingers. If the wrist is maintained in this position for too long, it becomes stiff. It is important that the athlete be educated to maintain ROM of the wrist and, when possible, hold the wrist in extension, especially while performing exercises. Optimal grip strength and ROM of the digits are accompanied by slight wrist extension. Also, the classic incorrect position of the hand and wrist during the healing phase includes slight wrist flexion, MP extension, and IP flexion. This is not functional in either sports or activities of daily living. This can be prevented by placing the injured hand in a wrist cock-up splint, especially at night, during the rehabilitation phase of recovery. The experienced therapist and trainer positions the digit with the MP joint in flexion and the IP joint in extension to prevent ligament contracture.

It is best for the hand to heal with MP joints extended and the IP joints flexed. It is also important when applying casts that the distal end of the cast or splint stops just proximal to the palmar crease of the volar surface of the hand, so that the splint does not prevent MP joint flexion and causes an extension contracture of the MP joint.

Strengthening exercises may begin at different times, depending on the type of injury and/or type of fixation, if surgery is necessary. Most patients with fractures and tendon injuries begin some form of strengthening at 4 to 6 weeks. To strengthen the muscle, resistance must be applied. Muscle tissue adapts to the amount of force placed upon it. There are several ways to do this in the hand and wrist. Resistive rubber bands, putty, dumbbells, and even manual resistance placed on the muscle by the therapist or athletic trainer can be used to overload the muscle. When ligaments of the wrist are injured or recovering from surgery, it is important to remember that traction forces placed upon these tissues are detrimental to tissue healing. A repaired scapholunate or lunotriquetral interosseous ligament should not have any traction forces placed upon it until about 12 weeks postoperatively. This key principle is important to the athletic

trainer or sports therapist to communicate with the strength coach to initiate strengthening exercises but to limit traction to the injured hand. Routine lifts in the weight room, such as the power clean, snatch and dead lift, are contraindicated for healing ligaments of the wrist. Other pitfalls in rehabilitation of the healing hand and wrist include allowing athletes to participate in plyometric or agility drills too soon. Box jumping and bag drills may not use the hand and wrist, but they do pose a risk for falling on the outstretched wrist, which may cause reinjury. Athletes should be given time for complete bone and soft tissue healing and to demonstrate strength that is near (within 85%) that of the noninvolved extremity. It is important to limit conditioning exercises in athletes with exposed Kirschner wires under casts, to decrease potential pin track infections.

PLAYING CASTS AND SPLINTS

The rules governing orthoses for competitive play vary with the specific sport, the level of play, and game official in charge of inspection and approval. Certain sports, such as swimming, wrestling, and (in some states) high school basketball, may not allow playing orthoses to be worn during competition (although they may be used during practice). A degree of uniformity for orthotic regulation has been attained in the rulebooks of the National Federation of State High School Association, the National Collegiate Athletic Association (NCAA), and the professional sports leagues.

In general, firm, but soft, plastics (consistency approximately that of a pencil eraser), such as RTV 11 (General Electric, Waterford, New York), a silicone-based paste applied in several layers alternating with gauze bandage wrapping, and Soft Cast (3M, Minneapolis, Minnesota) a preimpregnated gel roll, are popular, approved ingredients for construction of playing orthoses. Fiberglass or Gore-Tex may be used. Gore-Tex allows the patient to shower with the cast on. Prefabricated heat-malleable Plastazote splints have become popular. A layer of closed-cell polyurethane foam may be used to cover any of these orthoses during play or practice. This covering provides additional protection for the injured player and for opponents. For football, 0.25-inch-thick closed-cell foam is required in the National Football League, 0.5-inch in the NCAA, and 0.5-inch plus a physician's written letter or note of permission to play at the high school level (National Federation of High School Association rules since 1994).

In metacarpal fractures, flexion of the MP joints relaxes the intrinsic and extrinsic flexors, neutralizing their tendency to shorten and dorsally angulate the fractured metacarpal. The wrist may be positioned in 20° of extension. The MP joints may be left free or placed in 50° to 60° of flexion at the discretion of the treating physician. The IP joints usually are left free.

Buddy taping or splinting the injured finger to an adjacent finger prevents snagging and reinjury. The index finger is paired with the middle finger, the middle and ring finger are paired together (leaving the index finger free for writing and independent pinching), and the small finger is matched to the ring finger as closely as possible. For skill players (players that routinely handle the ball), the authors prefer to avoid taping across the flexor pads and finger joint creases to preserve sensation and finger flexion. For nonskill players, even the dominant hand may be covered completely with protective splint and padding.

RETURN TO PLAY

Return to play obviously varies from injury to injury. However, basic principles do apply. If fractures are present, the athlete should not be returned to play before callus formation has begun and there are minimal local symptoms such as edema. If a playing cast is worn over the injury, the athlete must be able to withstand a blow to the injured area.[8] Finally, if the injury involves collateral ligaments, three parameters must be taken into consideration. First, stability to the joint should not be compromised. If complete healing has not occurred, bracing or taping the joint for stability should be considered (**Fig. 4**). Second, acceptable ROM to successfully participate should be present. A lack of ROM decreases grip strength. Digits that do not have acceptable ROM will not be able to perform proper gripping, such as handling a racket, club, or bat. The inability to

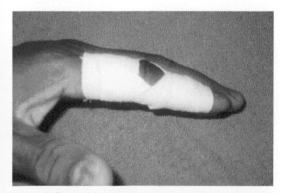

Fig. 4. Collateral ligament taping provides support for the collateral ligaments but allows the athlete to continue to flex and extend the digit for competition.

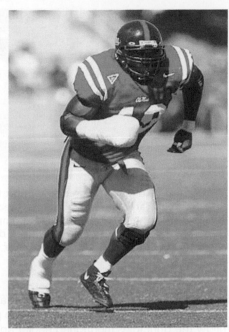

Fig. 5. The club cast is useful for nonskilled athletes for early return to competition. The concern is not reinjury to the athlete's original lesion, but to protect the digit from the high forces of grasping as compared with those of a direct blow. (*Courtesy of University of Mississippi Sports Information Department, University, MS; with permission.*)

grab and hold on to objects does not allow the injured athlete to perform such activities as tackling or catching. However, there are sports and positions in sports that allow for the wrist and hand to be completely covered in a cast and the athlete to still be able to participate. For example, in football, a linebacker or lineman can compete in what many athletic trainers refer to as a "club cast" (**Fig. 5**). For some fractures of the hand and wrist, the athletic trainer can position the injured wrist and/or hand so that the wrist is in slight extension and the MP joints and IP joints are flexed, so that the hand is placed somewhat in a full-fist position (**Fig. 6**). This does not allow for grasping objects with the digits but may allow for earlier return to play in the nonskilled positions in sports. A playing splint in the form of a properly padded short-arm cast, with the MP joints free, can provide limited gripping ability and perhaps allow for more skilled activities within sports. Metacarpal fractures that are nondisplaced and stable can often be treated in a short-arm cast with the injured metacarpal/finger taped to the adjacent finger. In this case, the injured finger is taped to the middle finger. The only time the index finger or the fifth finger should be buddy taped is if either of those fingers is actually injured. When

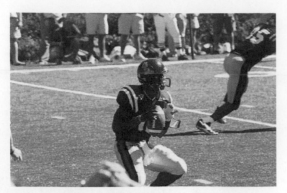

Fig. 6. Protective bracing may be used to support fractures of the metacarpophalangeal joint. Creative bracing allows the athlete to return early to competition but is able to limit reinjury to the involved digit. (*Courtesy of* Anna Burns, MD, ATC, University of Mississippi, University, MS.)

possible, the middle finger should be buddy taped with the ring finger. The key to a safe return to play is to follow the principles mentioned earlier and to choose the appropriate playing cast that allows for acceptable function with appropriate protection.

SUMMARY

Athletic injuries of the hand and wrist are common. Ideally, the key to management of these injuries is prevention. Athletes in certain sports and team positions are at a higher risk for injury to the fingers and wrists. Previously described bracing and taping techniques are useful to prevent injury.

Once injury occurs, rehabilitation of the hand and wrist is important. The fingers have a tendency to heal with the MP joints in extension and the IP joints flexed in the so-called "claw" position. The key is to brace the hand in the position of function, with MP joints flexed and the IP joints out straight,

to limit collateral ligament contracture. Once healing of the injured digit and wrist has occurred, rehabilitation of the injury is important. This requires close communication between the therapist and the strength and conditioning coach to allow strengthening exercises but to limit traction to the involved injury to limit the risk of reinjury.

Finally, once the injury has been rehabilitated, protective playing casts and splints are useful to allow the athlete to return early to competition and to decrease the risk of reinjury.

REFERENCES

1. Rettig AC, Wedenbener EJ, Gloyeske R, et al. Alternative management of mid-third scaphoid fractures in the athlete. Am J Sports Med 1994;22:711–4.
2. Beam J. Wrist. In: Fratantoro C, Abramowitz C, Pine JA, editors. Orthopedic taping, wrapping, bracing, padding. Philadelphia: F.A. Davis Company; 2006. p. 311–45.
3. Amadio PC. Epidemiology of hand and wrist injuries in sports. Hand Clin 1990;6:379–81.
4. Whiteside JA, Fleagle SB, Kalenak A, et al. Fractures and refractures in intercollegiate athletes. Am J Sports Med 1981;9:369–77.
5. Geissler WB. Carpal fractures in athletes. Arthroscopic surgery for the athletic elbow and wrist injuries. Clin Sports Med 2001;1(20):167–87.
6. Freeland A. Hand fractures: repair, reconstruction, and rehabilitation. Philadelphia: Churchill Livingstone; 2000. p. 67.
7. Norkin CC, Levangie PK. The hand and wrist complex. In: Joint structure and function. 2nd edition. Philadelphia: F.A. Davis Company; 1992. p. 274–7.
8. Rettig M. Wrist fractures in the athlete. Distal radius and carpal fractures. Clin Sports Med 1998;17(3): 469–89.

Index

Note: Page numbers of article titles are in **boldface** type.

A

Arthroscopic plication, in chronic posterolateral rotatory instability of elbow, 327–329

Arthroscopic reduction (Geissler technique), of scaphoid fractures, 364–370

Arthroscopy, in capitellar osteochondritis dessicans lesions, arthroscopic treatment of, 316, 318
in capsular contracture, 313
in fracture of elbow, 319
in fractures of capitellum, 319–321
in fractures of coronoid, 321
in management of scaphoid fractures, in athletes, **361–371**
in medial collateral ligament injury, 343–344
of elbow, complications of, 309–310
emerging role of, in chronic use injuries and fracture care, **307–323**
portal placement for, 307, 308
positions for, 307, 308
of radial head, 319
role in pain in medial elbow, 313–314

B

Baseball pitcher's elbow, reconstruction of medial collateral ligament, **341–348**

Biceps tendon, biomechanics of, 350
chronic ruptures of, surgical treatment of, 354
classification of, 350–351
complete rupture of, surgical treatment of, 352
injuries of, diagnosis of, 351–352
in athletes, **349–359**
surgical indications in, 352
surgical treatment of, 352–354
complications of, 355–356
postoperative regimen following, 354
results of, 355
partial ruptures of, surgical treatment of, 354
pathophysiology of, 350
surgical anatomy of, 349–350

Bony tunnel drilling, in medial collateral ligament injury, 344–345

Bracing, protective, for return to sport, 449, 450

C

Cage plate, for stabilization of metacarpal shaft fractures, 421

Capitate fractures, 402
complications of, 382–383
incidence of, 381
mechanism of injury in, 381
radiographic evaluation in, 381
treatment of, 382, 383

Capitellum, fractures of, arthroscopy in, 319–321

Capsular contracture, arthroscopy in, 313

Carpal fractures, in athletes, excluding scaphoid, **373–390**

Carpal ligament injury, and instability, 402–404
postoperative care following, 408

Carpus, anatomy of, 397
biomechanics of, 397–399
fracture(s) of, 400
percutaneous reduction of, 406–407
arthroscopic evaluation for, 407
screw fixation in, 407–408
injury of, diagnosis and workup in, 399
diagnostic imaging in, 400
in collision sports, 397, 398, 399
physical examination in, 399
instability of, management of, in athletes, **397–410**

Club cast, 418, 419, 449

Collateral ligament tears, 445

Condylar fractures, manual reduction of, 412
reduction under fluoroscopy, 412, 413

Coronoid, fractures of, arthroscopy in, 321

E

Elbow, anatomy of, 307
arthroscopy of, complications of, 309–310
emerging role of, in chronic use injuries and fracture care, **307–323**
portal placement for, 307, 308
positions for, 307, 308
distorted anatomy of, as contraindication to arthroscopy, 309
"drive-through" sign of, 327, 328
fracture of, arthroscopy in, 319
lateral, pain in, arthroscopic treatment of, 314
differential diagnosis of, 312
sawbones model of, 309
medial, pain in, role of arthroscopy in, 313–314
sawbones model of, 308, 309
medial collateral ligament of. See *Medial collateral ligament*.
posterior, sawbones model of, 309

Elbow (*continued*)
posterolateral rotatory instability of, 325
arthroscopic and open radial reconstruction of
ulnohumeral ligament for, **325–331**
arthroscopic repair in, 326–327, 328
chronic, arthroscopic plication in,
327–329
graft reconstruction of, open technique of,
329–330
hematoma in, 326
postoperative management of, 329
surgical reconstruction in, materials and
methods for, 330
results of, 330
surgical technique in, 326
sports-related injuries to, 309–310
topographic landmarks of, 307
Epicondylitis, lateral, 312, 313
conservative management of, 333–334
open and arthroscopic management of, in
athlete, **333–340**
operative treatment of, arthroscopic methods
of, 336, 337, 338
open methods of, 334–335
pathology of, 333
source of pain in, 333
Exercises, strengthening, following wrist and hand
injuries, 448
Extensor carpi radialis brevis, 333
anatomy of, 334
Extensor carpi radialis longus, anatomy of, 334

H

Hamate fractures, complications of, 379
examination in, 375, 376
imaging of, 376–377, 378
incidence of, 375
mechanism of injury in, 375
patterns of, 401–402
treatment of, 377–379
Hand, and wrist, injuries of, bracing and rehabilitation
for, in collegiate athletes, **445–450**
common, 445–446
prevention of, 446–447
rehabilitation following, 447–448
return to play following, 449
fractures of, 445
Headless cannulated screws, for fixation of
unicondylar fractures, 412
in unicondylar fractures of soft metaphysial bone,
413, 414
Headless mini screws, for fixation of phalangeal shaft
fractures, 416
Hematoma, in posterolateral rotatory instability of
elbow, 326

I

Interphalangeal joint, proximal. See *Proximal
interphalangeal joint*.

K

Kienböck disease, 402

L

Lag screw, for fixation of metacarpal shaft fractures,
420–421
Lateral collateral ligament, protection of, during
arthroscopy, 317–319
Lunate fractures, 402
complications of, 387
incidence of, 385
mechanism of injury in, 386
radiographic examination in, 386
treatment of, 386–387
Lunotriquetral ligament, instability, 403

M

McConnell arm positioner, 308
Medial collateral ligament, injury to, 311, 312
contact alterations due to, 312
history of, 342
imaging in, 343–344
physical examination in, 342–343
postoperative rehabilitation following, 346
treatment of, 344
surgical techniques for, 344–346, 347
pathophysiology of, 341–342
reconstruction of, in baseball pitcher's elbow,
341–348
Metacarpal fractures, and phalangeal fractures,
operative fixation of, goals of, 411
in athletes, **411–423**
Metacarpal head fractures, 419
fixation of, 419
Metacarpal shaft fractures, 419
cage plate stabilization of, 421
lag screw fixation of, 420–421
plate fixation of, 420
Metacarpophalangeal joint, of thumb, anatomy of,
439, 440
Metaphysial bone, soft, unicondylar fractures of,
headless cannulated screws in, 413, 414
MRI, in medial collateral ligament injury, 343
Muscle splitting, flexor-pronator origin, in medial
collateral ligament injury, 344

N

Neuritis, ulnar, 311–312

O

Osteochondritis dessicans, capitellar lesions,
        arthroscopic treatment of, 316, 318
            fixation and grafting of, 317, 318

P

Palmaris longus tendon grafts, in medial collateral
        ligament injury, 345
Perilunate dislocations, 403–404, 405
    closed reduction and percutaneous screw fixation
        in, 404, 405
Phalangeal base fractures, intraarticular, headless
        cannulated screws in, 414
Phalangeal fractures, and metacarpal fractures,
        operative fixation of, goals of, 411
            in athletes, **411–423**
Phalangeal shaft fractures, 415–418
    displaced, 415
    headless mini screw fixation in, 416
    plate fixation in, 415
Phalanx(ges), proximal, plate fixation of, 416–417,
        418, 419
            unicondylar fractures of, 412
            unicondylar fractures of, as unstable, 412
Pisiform fractures, 402
    complications of, 385
    incidence of, 384
    mechanism of injury in, 384
    radiographic examination in, 384, 385
Plates, for fixation of metacarpal shaft fractures,
        420
Playing casts, and splints, 448–449
Playing splint, specialized, 418
Proximal interphalangeal joint, anatomy of,
        425–426
    clinical features of, 429
    dislocations of, and fracture-dislocations of,
        treatment of, 429–430
        management of, in athletes, **425–437**
    dorsal, dislocations of, 426–427
            conservative management of, 430
    fracture-dislocations of, 427–429, 430
    imaging in, 429, 431
    injuries of, characteristics of, 426
    lateral, closed reduction of, 431
        dislocations of, 427, 428
        surgical repair of, 431
    management of, results and complications of,
        435–436
    open reduction internal fixation in, 433–435
    percutaneous pinning in, 431–432, 433
    skeletal traction in, 432–433
    sprains or complete tears of, 445
    volar, digital block and extension in, 431
        dislocations of, 427, 428

R

Radial head, arthroscopy of, 319
Radiocapitellar capsular complex, resection of,
        314–316, 317
Radiographs, plain, in medial collateral ligament
        injury, 343

S

Scaphoid, anatomy of, 397
    fixation of, guidewire placement for, 406
Scaphoid fractures, 398–399, 400
    acute nondisplaced, management of, 361
    arthroscopic management of, dorsal
        percutaneous approach for, 363–364
        in athletes, **361–371**
        indications for, 362
        preoperative evaluation for, 362–363
        surgical techniques in, 363–370
        volar percutaneous approach for, 363
    arthroscopic reduction of (Geissler technique),
        364–370
    displaced, open reduction and internal fixation of,
        361
    nonunion of, 398
    return to play following, 400, 401, 408
Scapholunate dissociation, 402
Scapholunate ligament, injury to, 402
        arthroscopy in, 402, 403
Splints, and playing casts, 448–449
    playing, specialized, 418
Sports-related injuries, to elbow, 309–310
Stener lesion, 440

T

Tennis elbow. See *Epicondylitis, lateral.*
Throwing, anatomy and biomechanics of, 310–311
Throwing athlete, elbow pathology in, arthroscopic
        treatment of, 314
Thumb, metacarpophalangeal joint of, anatomy of,
        439, 440
Trapezium fractures, complications of, 380
    examination in, 380
    incidence of, 379
    mechanism of injury in, 380
    radiographic evaluation in, 380
    treatment of, 380
Trapezoid fractures, complications of, 384
    incidence of, 383
    mechanism of injury in, 383
    radiographic evaluation in, 384
    treatment of, 384
Triangular fibrocartilage complex, tears of,
    arthroscopic evaluation of, 392–393
        arthroscopic repair of, complications of, 395

Triangular (*continued*)
  imaging findings for, 392
  in athletes, **391–396**
  operative indications for, 392
  operative technique for, 393–395
  postoperative course following, 395
  preoperative evaluation for, 392
Triquetral fractures, 400–401
  complications of, 375
  examination in, 373–374
  incidence of, 373
  mechanism of injury in, 373, 374
  radiographic evaluation of, 374
  treatment of, 374–375

U

Ulnar collateral ligament(s), acute injury of, 440
  diagnosis of, 440–441
  in athlete, **439–444**
  pattern of, 440
  treatment of, 441–443
  anatomy of, 439, 440
Ulnar nerve handling, in medial collateral ligament
    injury, 344
Ulnar neuritis, 311–312
Ulnohumeral ligament, arthroscopic and open radial
    reconstruction of, for posterolateral rotatory
    instability of elbow, **325–331**
Ultrasonography, in medial collateral ligament injury,
    343
Unicondylar fractures, headless cannulated screw
    fixation of, 414–415

of phalanges, as unstable, 412
of proximal phalanx, 412
  headless cannulated miniscrew fixation in,
      412
of soft metaphysial bone, headless cannulated
    screws in, 413, 414
types of, 411

V

Valgus stress test, 333

W

Wrist. See also *Carpus*.
  and hand, injuries of, bracing and rehabilitation
      for, in collegiate athletes, **445–450**
      common, 445–446
      prevention of, 446–447
      rehabilitation following, 449
      return to play following, 449
  diagnostic arthroscopy of, and percutaneous
      reduction and fixation techniques, 404–406
      preparation for, 406
  injury of, prevention of, 404
  sprains of, 446
  taping of, to prevent injury, 446–447

X

"X" technique, taping of wrist, 446

Printed and bound by CPI Group (UK) Ltd, Croydon, CR0 4YY

03/10/2024

01040348-0017